WALL PILATES WORKOUTS FOR WOMEN

THE ULTIMATE 30-DAY BODY TRANSFORMATION PLAN TO
TONE YOUR GLUTES, BACK & ABS AND BOOST STRENGTH,
BALANCE, AND FLEXIBILITY
(COMPLETE WITH EASY-TO-FOLLOW ILLUSTRATIONS)

Miranda Rosewood

© Copyright 2024 by Miranda Rosewood - All rights reserved.

The content contained within this book may not be reproduced, duplicated or transmitted without direct written permission from the author or the publisher.

Under no circumstances will any blame or legal responsibility be held against the publisher, or author, for any damages, reparation, or monetary loss due to the information contained within this book, either directly or indirectly.

Legal Notice:

This book is copyright protected. It is only for personal use. You cannot amend, distribute, sell, use, quote or paraphrase any part, or the content within this book, without the consent of the author or publisher.

Disclaimer Notice:

Please note the information contained within this document is for educational and entertainment purposes only. All effort has been executed to present accurate, up to date, reliable, complete information. No warranties of any kind are declared or implied. Readers acknowledge that the author is not engaged in the rendering of legal, financial, medical or professional advice. The content within this book has been derived from various sources. Please consult a licensed professional before attempting any techniques outlined in this book.

By reading this document, the reader agrees that under no circumstances is the author responsible for any losses, direct or indirect, that are incurred as a result of the use of the information contained within this document, including, but not limited to, errors, omissions, or inaccuracies.

...ODUCTION

...ongest time, I made excuses for my fitness (or lack thereof), citing not having time to ...e gym as one of the core reasons. I am sure you can relate to how hectic life can get for ...omen, juggling our time between family, career, and trying to have a life! I had to make ...al decision to take my health into my own hands and, by so doing, I discovered that I ...ing I need to stay fit without needing to go to the gym. So many other people have also ... realization, and there is a wealth of resources online that will give you more reasons to ... Ensuring you are active for at least 30 minutes per day can make a significant difference ...ss, without any extra equipment needed. Walking through your neighborhood or dancing ... video on YouTube can give you all the cardio you need to stay strong and healthy. You ... your body weight to build strength through planks, push-ups, and exercises that target ...scle groups (C, 2023). In this guide, we will explore the effectiveness of home exercises to ... your fitness goals, with a focus on wall Pilates. These exercises have a low barrier of entry ...erefore easy to get started with right away.

...he age of technology and the internet, there is a plethora of resources available, such ..., that enable you to work out in the comfort of your own home. I am particularly drawn ...roach because I struggle to feel comfortable working out in front of strangers, especially ...'t feel like I am in my best shape. Furthermore, staying consistent with my workouts can ... if my fitness routine involves an additional commute. As a result, I usually drop the habit ...t very far with it, even when I'm paying for an expensive membership! It can also be tricky ... figure out the mechanisms of some gym equipment, and there isn't always anyone available ...ith this guide, you can be confident about your safety during workouts. There will be clear, ...ollow steps that also highlight key aspects to watch out for, helping you to maintain correct ...e exercising. Furthermore, you can track your progress in a section provided later in the ...ch will motivate you to persist in your fitness journey.

... many types of workouts you can choose to engage in for an effective home-based routine, ...mportant to mix things up and touch on all areas of your body. Make sure to include cardio ...outine, which you can factor in through jogging, walking, or aerobics. Your strength-training ... should be divided between your lower and upper body to ensure you are targeting all the ... in your body; wall Pilates is the perfect method for this, especially when you are in a time ...n many ways, it is the best of both worlds, as it provides the perfect intensity that targets ... most women are particular about in their fitness journeys. Pilates has changed my life and ...ew fitness, and I am happy to be sharing this knowledge with you too—and excited for the ...ahead!

Table of CONTENTS

Introduction	6
Chapter 1: Pilates Fundamentals	8
What Is Wall Pilates?	8
Tracing Its Origins	8
Is Wall Pilates Worth the Hype?	9
Wall Pilates During Pregnancy: Is It Safe?	11
Chapter 2: Understanding the Core Principles	12
The Six Core Pillars of Pilates Explained	12
The Magic of the Mind–Body Connection	13
Chapter 3: Setting the Stage	16
The Tools of the Trade	16
Practicing Wall Pilates at Home	17
Chapter 4: Stronger by the Wall	21
Wall Push-Ups	21
Wall Squats	24
High Lunge Pose Against the Wall	26
Wall Sphinx Pose	28
Wall Bridge	30
Wall Handstand	32
Wall Plank	34
Chapter 5: Boosting Stamina With Wall Workouts	36
Wall Mountain Climbers	36
Wall Sit	38
Wall Lunges	40
Wall Burpees	42

Wall Scissor Kicks

Wall Bicycle Crunches

Wall Sit With Leg Lifts

Chapter 6: Enhancing Stability With Wall Pilates

Wall Angels

Wall Dead Bug

Wall Slides

Wall Clock

Wall Side Plank

Wall Pike Push-Ups

Wall Lean Toe Lifts

Wall Russian Twists

Wall Staff Pose

Side-Lying Wall Leg Lift

Chapter 7: Wall Pilates for Supreme Flexibility

Legs-Up-The-Wall

Wall Downward Facing Dog

Hamstring Stretch in Doorway

Wall Shoulder Stand

Wall Half Happy Baby Pose

Wall Garland Pose (Back to Wall)

Forward Fold Against Wall

Wall Camel Pose With Strap

Wall Soleus Stretch

Gastroc Stretch on Wall

Wall Chest Stretch

Chapter 8: 30 Days to a Healthier, Stronger You

Track Your Progress

References

INTRODUCTION

For the longest time, I made excuses for my fitness (or lack thereof), citing not having time to go to the gym as one of the core reasons. I am sure you can relate to how hectic life can get for us as women, juggling our time between family, career, and trying to have a life! I had to make an intentional decision to take my health into my own hands and, by so doing, I discovered that I have everything I need to stay fit without needing to go to the gym. So many other people have also come to this realization, and there is a wealth of resources online that will give you more reasons to believe this. Ensuring you are active for at least 30 minutes per day can make a significant difference in your fitness, without any extra equipment needed. Walking through your neighborhood or dancing to a Zumba video on YouTube can give you all the cardio you need to stay strong and healthy. You can also use your body weight to build strength through planks, push-ups, and exercises that target specific muscle groups (C, 2023). In this guide, we will explore the effectiveness of home exercises to accomplish your fitness goals, with a focus on wall Pilates. These exercises have a low barrier of entry and are therefore easy to get started with right away.

Thanks to the age of technology and the internet, there is a plethora of resources available, such as this one, that enable you to work out in the comfort of your own home. I am particularly drawn to this approach because I struggle to feel comfortable working out in front of strangers, especially when I don't feel like I am in my best shape. Furthermore, staying consistent with my workouts can be difficult if my fitness routine involves an additional commute. As a result, I usually drop the habit before I get very far with it, even when I'm paying for an expensive membership! It can also be tricky to try and figure out the mechanisms of some gym equipment, and there isn't always anyone available to help. With this guide, you can be confident about your safety during workouts. There will be clear, easy-to-follow steps that also highlight key aspects to watch out for, helping you to maintain correct form while exercising. Furthermore, you can track your progress in a section provided later in the book, which will motivate you to persist in your fitness journey.

There are many types of workouts you can choose to engage in for an effective home-based routine, and it is important to mix things up and touch on all areas of your body. Make sure to include cardio in your routine, which you can factor in through jogging, walking, or aerobics. Your strength-training workouts should be divided between your lower and upper body to ensure you are targeting all the muscles in your body; wall Pilates is the perfect method for this, especially when you are in a time crunch. In many ways, it is the best of both worlds, as it provides the perfect intensity that targets the areas most women are particular about in their fitness journeys. Pilates has changed my life and how I view fitness, and I am happy to be sharing this knowledge with you too—and excited for the journey ahead!

Wall Scissor Kicks	44
Wall Bicycle Crunches	46
Wall Sit With Leg Lifts	48
Chapter 6: Enhancing Stability With Wall Pilates	51
Wall Angels	51
Wall Dead Bug	54
Wall Slides	56
Wall Clock	58
Wall Side Plank	60
Wall Pike Push-Ups	62
Wall Lean Toe Lifts	64
Wall Russian Twists	66
Wall Staff Pose	68
Side-Lying Wall Leg Lift	70
Chapter 7: Wall Pilates for Supreme Flexibility	72
Legs-Up-The-Wall	72
Wall Downward Facing Dog	74
Hamstring Stretch in Doorway	74
Wall Shoulder Stand	78
Wall Half Happy Baby Pose	80
Wall Garland Pose (Back to Wall)	82
Forward Fold Against Wall	84
Wall Camel Pose With Strap	86
Wall Soleus Stretch	88
Gastroc Stretch on Wall	90
Wall Chest Stretch	92
Chapter 8: 30 Days to a Healthier, Stronger You	94
Track Your Progress	109
References	**114**

Table of CONTENTS

Introduction	6
Chapter 1: Pilates Fundamentals	8
What Is Wall Pilates?	8
Tracing Its Origins	8
Is Wall Pilates Worth the Hype?	9
Wall Pilates During Pregnancy: Is It Safe?	11
Chapter 2: Understanding the Core Principles	12
The Six Core Pillars of Pilates Explained	12
The Magic of the Mind-Body Connection	13
Chapter 3: Setting the Stage	16
The Tools of the Trade	16
Practicing Wall Pilates at Home	17
Chapter 4: Stronger by the Wall	21
Wall Push-Ups	21
Wall Squats	24
High Lunge Pose Against the Wall	26
Wall Sphinx Pose	28
Wall Bridge	30
Wall Handstand	32
Wall Plank	34
Chapter 5: Boosting Stamina With Wall Workouts	36
Wall Mountain Climbers	36
Wall Sit	38
Wall Lunges	40
Wall Burpees	42

You don't just have to take my word for it when it comes to the effectiveness of Pilates. Many women speak openly about how Pilates has changed their bodies and made them stronger and leaner in a shorter time compared with workout regimes that focus mostly on cardio, for example. Celebrities such as Lady Gaga, Miley Cyrus, and Cameron Diaz, to name a few, also rave about Pilates as an effective and convenient workout that not only allows you to achieve your body goals but also improves your posture and aids in alleviating chronic back pain, among other things (Bell, 2023). So, let that amp up your energy and motivation to begin your own transformative Pilates journey!

Until now, it would have been very difficult to find all the information you need about wall Pilates—from the health benefits to tips for best practices—in one place. But I have created this guide to be your one-stop shop for all things wall Pilates. I chose to focus on wall-assisted exercises specifically because they are beginner-friendly; they also allow you to build up your strength and try different variations to cater to your body's needs and abilities. There is also minimal equipment required, which makes these exercises accessible and reduces your resistance to getting going.

This book is structured as a 30-day challenge to give you a clear goal to work toward, but also one that is achievable and realistic regardless of your fitness level. By the time you reach day 30, you will be able to see the results of your efforts, which will empower you to continue on this incredible path of taking care of yourself and prioritizing your fitness.

Let's dive in!

CHAPTER 1
STRONGER PILATES FUNDAMENTALS

I imagine you are ready to dig in and start working on your fitness goals. However, it is important to start by getting all the fundamentals down. A firm foundation is necessary if you plan on building a habit that lasts and an exercise routine that works and is effective. As famous basketball player Michael Jordan once said, "Get the fundamentals down and the level of everything you do will rise" (Jordan, n.d).

What Is Wall Pilates?

Wall Pilates became trendy on the social media platform TikTok in early 2023, but it has been around for much longer than that. It is simply Pilates done with wall support, offering resistance that would normally come from a fancy reformer machine or gym equipment. You lean your back, side, arms, or feet on the wall, and that resistance, coupled with your body weight, can give you a full, intense, and effective workout (Porter, 2023). Let's look into the history of Pilates and how it has evolved, before we dive into the benefits of wall Pilates and why it has become so popular.

Tracing Its Origins

Pilates was created in the 1920s by Germans Joseph and Clara Pilates, who initially designed it as a rehabilitation method for injury recovery. Joseph had served as a hospital orderly during World War I, during which time he tried his methods with patients who could not walk. This is when he first developed what is now known as the reformer machine, which was then known as "the Cadillac." Later, he and his wife moved to New York, where they opened the first Pilates studio Pilates quickly grew in popularity among the dance and theater communities as they discovered that it rehabilitated them back to normal after injury more quickly than other methods. They also realized it improved their performance and form. News of it spread quickly and attracted the attention of celebrities and other famous people, who would go to New York to see it for themselves (About Pilates, n.d.).

The reformer machine uses a spring tension and pulley machine to provide resistance, which aids in strength training and helps bring your body back into proper form and alignment by strengthening your core muscles. Fun fact: Originally, Pilates was called "Contrology," and Joseph and Clara shared their teachings by co-authoring a book, Return to Life Through Contrology. It only took on the name "Pilates" after Joseph died in 1967. Today, much of the equipment used, although modern, is heavily based on what was introduced by Joseph and Clara nine decades ago (About Pilates, n.d.). And with new knowledge and modifications, the same exercises can be done with only a mat, your weight, and, as you will learn later in this book, a wall!

Is Wall Pilates Worth the Hype?

To be direct, yes—wall Pilates lives up to the hype! You can find countless testimonies of people who have seen great results and swear by this exercise type. The benefits are so far-reaching that we could have an entire book just on this topic, so here we will focus on just a few of the ones that will get you amped up to get started (Mukhwana, 2023b).

Accessibility

All you need to get started is a wall. There is no barrier to entry, as is the case with joining a costly Pilates studio or buying the machines for your home. Besides, most people don't have the space for all that bulky equipment. You also won't end up procrastinating until you have bought a membership or equipment, because you will already have all you need: your weight and a wall.

Increased Core Strength and Function

The core muscles support much of the body and are critical in helping us maintain stability and balance. Wall Pilates targets all the core muscles, namely the abdominals, obliques, hips, and lower back, instead of just the abs, which is the case with most core exercises. A strong core is a vital part of fitness and maintaining an overall healthy body, and this workout saves you time and energy by targeting all the muscles at once.

Relief From Back Pain

If you experience back pain, this may be related to bad posture and your spine not being aligned. Because both of these issues are addressed in wall Pilates, one of the direct benefits is relief from back pain. The muscles that support the spine are also strengthened by this form of exercise, which leaves you with a more upright and lengthened posture.

Improved Spinal Alignment

The extremely sedentary lifestyle that most people have means that you probably spend much of your time hunched over a desk or laptop. In addition, as we grow older, our spines experience many changes and develop more curvature over time. The resulting compressed and curved spine affects our posture and spinal alignment. Wall Pilates aids in dealing with this problem as it lengthens the spine and strengthens the glutes, abs, and back muscles, which help support the spine.

Energy Boost

Wall Pilates encompasses smooth, controlled movements that do not leave you feeling extremely tired but still increase your cardiorespiratory capacity—in other words, it increases your blood circulation and oxygen flow. There is also the release of feel-good hormones (endorphins), which also boost your energy.

Lower Risk of Injury

Injury often comes from strained muscles or joint pain because of poor mobility or a lack of strength in muscles that the body relies on for support. Wall Pilates tackles all three of these factors, improving your flexibility, mobility, and strength, leaving you less susceptible to the injuries and body aches and pains that result from a lack of exercise.

Enhanced Proprioception

Proprioception is your ability to determine your body's position in space and time at any point. It allows you to walk without looking at your feet the entire time, or to touch any part of your body with your eyes closed. Proprioception is essential to maintain your balance, especially if you do active sports or work an active job where you are moving around a lot. Wall Pilates enhances proprioception because the movements require you to move into different planes in a smooth, controlled, but quick manner, which enhances your balance.

Stress Relief

Wall Pilates releases endorphins, which play a role in regulating our mood and making us feel good. The active movements and physical exertion lead to tension release not only in the muscles but also in the mind. Be intentional about breathing deeply while working out, as this will also leave you feeling lighter and happier when you are done (breathing correctly also increases the effectiveness of exercise in general).

Better Flexibility and Mobility

Flexibility is how much your muscles can stretch and extend, while mobility is the range of motion in your joints, such as your hips, knees, and shoulders. Your mobility level is dependent on your strength and flexibility, both of which are enhanced by wall Pilates.

Relief From Menstrual Pain

By targeting the pelvis and lower back muscles, wall Pilates is said to help with menstrual pain. Inflammation is also reduced because of the increased blood circulation in the larger muscle groups (Mukhwana, 2023b).

Wall Pilates During Pregnancy: Is It Safe?

If you are pregnant, you will be happy to know that wall Pilates is safe during pregnancy. Of course, it is always wise to consult your doctor before you begin. One of the main components that makes it safe is the wall support, as well as the adaptability of the workouts. Pilates is also generally easy on the joints and relieves common pains faced during pregnancy, such as back pain. You can increase or decrease the intensity of the movements according to how you feel and how far along you are in your pregnancy. Wall Pilates can be highly beneficial in pregnancy because it strengthens the muscles used during labor. The cardiorespiratory benefits also aid in calming your mind and relaxing your body, as well as preparing your mind and endurance for delivery. Your growing baby also benefits from exercise, as it stimulates brain development and prevents susceptibility to some illnesses (Menzies, 2021).

Summary

Now that we have laid the foundation about what wall Pilates is, where it came from, and how it benefits the body, we can now continue to look in more detail at the core principles of Pilates. This will ensure that when you start the 30-day challenge, you will be well-equipped to maintain the correct form and focus on what is important to achieve the results you want to see.

CHAPTER 2
UNDERSTANDING THE CORE PRINCIPLES

Committing fully to anything in life requires an understanding of its fundamental principles. The same is true for exercise. In our case, understanding what makes wall Pilates effective will motivate you further on your fitness journey, meaning your chances of seeing the 30-day challenge through will be greatly increased. Knowing the why behind an action you commit to can be summed up in these words by Judith Guest, American novelist and screenwriter: "To have a reason to get up in the morning, it is necessary to have some kind of guiding principle. A belief of some kind" (Guest, n.d). The feeling and certainty described in this quote is what I am aiming to provide for you in this chapter, so that when you wake up each morning you are motivated to take on the challenge because you know you will get the results you want. Let's dive right in.

The Six Core Pillars of Pilates Explained

To experience the full benefits of Pilates, you must perform all the exercises correctly, paying close attention to the core principles of the exercises (The 10 Principles of Pilates, 2020).

Breathing

Correct breathing in Pilates is important, as it allows you to properly engage your inner abdominal muscles. This relieves tension in places that shouldn't be tense, specifically your neck and back. Breathing properly also enables efficient blood circulation to your muscles, providing a much-needed oxygen supply. While practicing wall Pilates, you should ensure that your breathing is aligned with your body movements, inhaling as you relax your muscles and exhaling as you contract them.

Concentration

Concentrating on each movement as you complete an exercise ensures you are engaging the correct muscle group and maintaining the correct form. You can do this by mindfully visualizing the targeted muscles as you breathe through the movements. This also allows the rest of your body to be in the correct alignment to fully support the movement you are performing. Concentration also stimulates your brain and neuromuscular system to cooperate allowing you to get the most out of each movement.

Centering

Centering involves engaging what Joseph Pilates termed "the powerhouse" of Pilates, which is the abdominal muscles, lower back, gluteal muscles, and hips. Performing movements with a focus on these muscles being engaged enhances your core strength, allowing you to progress in your Pilates journey. This also enhances your quality of life, as it improves your posture, balance, and stability as well.

Control

Control was the epicenter of Pilates at its inception, which is why it was first known as "Contrology." Pilates requires each movement to be precise and deliberate, not random or unstructured. You should also move through each movement slowly, squeezing and contracting each muscle carefully. With wall Pilates, the extra support makes some movements easier while also providing more resistance; these controlled movements lead to enhanced strengthening of your muscles.

Precision

Precision is a step further into control and concentration, where each singular movement is seen not as a means to an end but as purposeful in and of itself. The more you practice Pilates, the more you will notice that you can identify any errors in form and alignment that you need to correct. Working with the support of a wall also allows you to see which side of your body is weaker and which areas need more work. Precision also allows you to pay attention to the nuanced aspects of Pilates and ensure that every inch of your body is engaged.

Flow

Pilates must be performed gracefully, with a smooth and continuous flow between movements. Don't be discouraged if, at first, this does not occur easily. With practice, you will master the movements and become more seamless in your execution of them.

As you can tell, all of these principles work together to create an effective exercise routine. Being mindful throughout will enable you to pay attention to these details and, with good guidance, you will receive reminders of what to pay attention to for each movement, as you will see with the exercises outlined in this guide. Let's dive deeper into the aspect of concentration and explore the mind–body connection.

The Magic of the Mind–Body Connection

Neuroscientific studies have proven that the parts of our brain that are activated while doing an activity are also activated when we visualize the movement with deep concentration. This phenomenon is known as "mental rehearsal" or "motor imagery," and has also been proven to enhance performance for athletes. This can be attributed to the fact that the parts of our brain responsible for planning, execution, and coordination of the movement are all activated, and, with practice, this improves our actual execution of said movement (Ladda et al., 2021). Imagine coupling this visualization with performing a movement—this is essentially what the mind–body connection is all about.

One of the more popular quotes from Joseph Pilates is, "Pilates is a complete coordination of mind, body and soul" (What Is the Mind-Body Connection in Pilates?, 2018). This is one of the key elements that sets Pilates apart from other exercises. The results that people often get with Pilates are markedly different from what they'd see if they spent the same amount of time going to the gym, for example, because of the emphasis on working with the mind to achieve results. Everything begins in the mind, leading to a better awareness of how movements are executed, which engages the inner muscles and improves overall execution. This leads to better results. The mind–body connection marries the core pillars of Pilates that we discussed earlier to create an effective exercise (How the Pilates Mind–Body Connection Works for You, n.d.).

The Effects

Increased Mental Sharpness

As you move through the Pilates movements with precision and concentration, your neural pathways are stimulated, enhancing your mental sharpness and clarity. Your cognitive focus is sharpened because of the concentration required when engaging with the mind–body connection. Coordination is required to execute Pilates movements properly, and concentration also enhances this function of the brain. Concentration also contributes to the brain's neuroplasticity, which is when the brain reorganizes itself while forming new neural connections. This process also contributes to the enhanced cognitive function of the brain (How the Pilates Mind–Body Function Works for You, 2022).

Increased Body Awareness

Due to the deep concentration afforded by the mind–body connection, you have to pay close attention to how your body moves. This increases awareness of muscular function and detects which areas need more attention to increase strength and stability. Your proprioception, which is your body's ability to sense its position in time and space, is also improved as you become more attuned to your body movements. You also gain a deeper understanding and appreciation of your body's capabilities and limitations, allowing you to make changes and adjustments where necessary to get the most out of your workouts (The Mind Body Connection: Key Elements in Pilates, Part 3, n.d.).

Increased Positive Focus

Dedicating time to Pilates can also improve your mental well-being through mindfulness. Removing your focus from possible negative triggers and emotions will leave you feeling better after your workout. In addition, being able to complete a Pilates workout with mindfulness will give you a sense of accomplishment, which enhances the mental positive reinforcement that can be beneficial both on and off the mat (How the Pilates Mind–Body Function Works for You, 2022).

Reduced Stress

Pilates has a strong focus not only on mindfulness while practicing but also on breathing, as we have already discussed. When these two are coupled, it activates the parasympathetic nervous system, thus promoting relaxation. A direct result of this is stress management. This also leads to the release of hormones called endorphins, which put you in a good mood and leave you feeling great after a workout. This is why, regardless of how you felt when you started, you will always end any workout feeling good, positive, and optimistic (How the Pilates Mind–Body Function Works for You, 2022).

Summary

From what we have seen in this chapter, Pilates is a unique exercise that takes care of not only our physical fitness but our mental fitness as well. When you begin the exercises, remember to align yourself with the core principles of Pilates. Take deep inhales and exhales, concentrating fully on how your body moves through each movement. Keep your movements slow, deliberate, and specific while maintaining the proper alignment. Harness the mind-body connection to see even better results from your workouts.

Now that we have the technical aspects figured out, we will consider some helpful information and tips to ensure your Pilates journey is smooth, safe, and fun!

CHAPTER 3
UNDERSTANDING SETTING THE STAGE

Imagine going on a road trip on an unfamiliar trail with no map, GPS, or friend who knows the way! In the wise words of Yogi Berra, "If you don't know where you are going, you'll end up someplace else," (Berra, n.d). This chapter is dedicated to giving you a road map before you start the ultimate 30-day wall Pilates challenge. To ensure your success, you need the background knowledge (which you now have) and the directions that will enable you to embark on your wall Pilates journey with confidence. Let's first consider the things you need.

The Tools of the Trade

A distinctive aspect of wall Pilates lies in its accessible nature ,characterized by an exceptionally low barrier to entry .It doesn't matter if you have a small space—all you need is an empty space in your home next to a wall and you're good to go .However ,there are a few things you can add to make your workouts even more effective and comfortable:

- **A mat:** This offers you a comfortable platform so you are cushioned from the cold, hard floor. It also offers extra support, which protects you from injuries.

- **An open wall space:** You must ensure that the space you choose is free of any hazards that may trip you or that you can hit your hand or foot against. Clear away any furniture so you can comfortably jump jacks and do snow angels with no obstructions in the way. Also, ensure the wall is smooth and flat.

- **A soft cushion for support:** You may need an extra layer of protection and support, which you can get from a cushion. This will also help with alignment and protect you from injuries. There are also some movements where much of your body is in the air, so it is a good idea to have something comfortable to fall back on.

Choosing the Right Pilates Mat

Picking a mat from the many available options can be quite tricky .Let's consider what makes a great mat for wall Pilates.

There are some key aspects to consider when buying a Pilates mat, because it is meant to cushion your spine and bony joints—in comparison to a yoga mat, for example, which enables you to stand with balance) *Choosing the Right Pilates Mat:(2017,*

- **Thickness:** The recommended thickness is between 8mm and 15 mm, as this offers enough support and alignment. A 6mm mat is a decent compromise, especially if you need to use the mat for other workouts as well.

- **Material:** You need to ensure the mat supports a good grip and prevents you from slipping and sliding, which can cause serious injury. Cork mats are a fantastic option as they come with the added advantage of being antimicrobial and nontoxic, offering a sustainable solution.

- **Size:** When it comes to your mat, size does matter! Some movements require you to lie down completely, rolling over and extending your body lengthwise. You must ensure that your head and feet remain protected to avoid injuries. Opt for the longest mat you can find.

- **Durability:** Again, thinking about sustainability, it is better to invest in a mat that will last for a long time than one you will need to keep replacing.

- **Portability:** A mat that you can carry around easily comes in handy. You may decide to attend a live session with others and, for hygiene purposes, it is always good to take your own mat. You can also switch things up and exercise in different areas of the house when you get bored of the scenery in one room. If you can get a mat with a shoulder strap, even better! That way, you can live out your Pilates mom fantasy (with the full gear we will detail in a moment).

Practicing Wall Pilates at Home

As with any exercises done at home, it is important that we go over some points on how to proceed with caution. Because there is no instructor to keep an eye on your form and alignment, injuries can occur. But, of course, there are things you can do to progress safely.

Let's start by going over some possible questions you may have regarding who can do wall Pilates. As already covered, wall Pilates is perfectly safe to practice during pregnancy. It is also ideal for people who are experiencing back pain and those who may be recovering from injury, as it can help with regaining strength and building muscle as you nurse yourself back to health. Seniors with limited mobility can also practice wall Pilates. This is recommended because of the additional support this exercise provides (Mukhwana, 2023b).

Next, let's consider some do's and dont's to ensure you exercise safely. Always begin and end your workouts with a warm-up and cool-down session. This protects you from injuries and warms up the muscles targeted by workouts. You should also ensure proper, deep breathing, keeping a relaxed rib cage.

Also keep your arms, neck, and shoulders relaxed while maintaining a straight back to guard against injury. It is also better to have shorter sessions spread across the week than to cram everything into one hour per week. Lastly, remember to keep your core engaged throughout the session (Ward, 2019).

Never hold your breath while doing Pilates! Breathing, as already discussed, is an important aspect of doing the movements correctly. You should also never try to do too much too soon as this may lead to injury if you overstretch or try to force your body into a movement you are not yet comfortable with. Your flexibility will improve gradually, so be patient and take your time. Avoid having your stomach muscles relaxed and bulging outward, rotating your pelvis. Don't hesitate to use a soft cushion for your back and neck, especially when you are just starting and if you feel pain in these areas while working out (Jacob, 2020).

With the important admin out of the way, it's time to go shopping!

What to Wear

Choosing the correct gear for your workout will make it much more enjoyable and easier, as your clothing will not be in the way. For wall Pilates, it is best to wear form-fitting clothing—as you will be contorting your body into different shapes, you need to be able to do so without obstructions. It is also a good idea to wear socks with grip pads on the bottom to prevent slipping during your workout. A sports bra is recommended for extra support, although wall Pilates is relatively low impact. That's about it! Simple and straightforward, and you're ready to go (Edna, 2019).

The Four S's of Wall Pilates

We will now do a quick run-through of what to expect in the 30-day challenge, and what exercises are outlined in the rest of this book.

Pilates represents a functional fitness approach designed to boost fitness and mobility by emphasizing the integration and refinement of the four S's: strength, stamina, stretch, and stability. Wall Pilates encompasses all of these aspects within its exercises. In this section, we will briefly introduce how wall Pilates effectively targets these four areas. In the upcoming chapters, you can look forward to exploring each one in greater detail as you embark on your exercise journey, delving into exercises specific to the four facets outlined below (Turnquist, n.d.):

- **Strength** can be divided into three categories: core, upper body, and lower body. Some exercises target a specific aspect of strength, but you will find that Pilates often targets multiple muscle groups even if your focus is on one. For example, exercises to strengthen your core will often also target your hip flexors and hamstring muscles. Pilates requires consistency for you to have long and lean muscles. It uses low-impact exercises to achieve results versus higher-impact exercises such as weightlifting.

- **Stamina** is a measure of your endurance, or how long you can keep doing the same exercise without stopping. You will discover throughout your journey that, with practice, your stamina will improve as your core strengthens and your fitness level improves.

- **Stability** is your ability to maintain a straight back and remain rooted to your center while you move your other limbs in all directions. As a beginner you may struggle with this, but don't despair! Stability relies on your powerhouse—that is, your core strength. As you strengthen your core, you will become more stable and move through more exercises easily.

- **Stretching** focuses on your flexibility and how far you can extend your limbs away from your body comfortably. For example, if you are sitting up straight, how far can you reach to touch your feet? This is a simple way to check your flexibility and track your progress. As you start, you may barely be able to reach your knees, but you will discover that after a few weeks your hands begin to inch closer to your feet, if they're not already touching them! Stretching should not be ignored—include it at the end of your workouts when you are cooling down.

Summary

You will soon learn that wall Pilates is a form of exercise that is rewarding and fulfilling. Additionally, you are now well-equipped to get started as we have discussed what you need, what to wear, and how to exercise safely. The following four chapters will detail exercises that focus on each of the four S's in turn.

Watercooler Conversations

"Take care of your body .It's the only place you have to live – ".Jim Rohn

How many watercooler conversations have you had with other women about the struggle to fit exercise into daily life? I can tell you, I've had many. Our time is split between family responsibilities and our careers – and if we're lucky, maybe even a bit of a social life too!

What's worse is that there's always one lady in the office who somehow manages to do it all... She's been to the gym and she's already sitting at her desk sipping her smoothie when you get to work. We all want to know her secret – yet none of us need it.

When I realized I had everything I needed to stay in shape without setting foot in the gym, it transformed my life... Specifically, wall Pilates transformed my life.

So the next time you find yourself in one of those office conversations with someone who feels terrible about their fitness and is struggling to think of ways to fit exercise into their routine, tell them about how much there is they can do at home. Better yet, give them a copy of this book – then they'll have everything they need to get started.

You can extend that help to women you'll never even meet in person too. All you have to do is leave a short review.

By leaving a review of this book on Amazon, you'll shine a light on the path for other women who are desperate to improve their fitness quickly and easily.

You can guarantee that many people are looking for a solution this simple and straightforward, and your review will help them find it. The result? Fewer miserable ladies at the watercooler!

Thank you so much for your support. We need all the help we can get in this busy world!

CHAPTER 4
STRONGER BY THE WALL

The first thing we will focus on is developing the powerhouse—your core. As you have already learned, this is the main aspect governing your success with wall Pilates. As you progress through the exercises, remember these encouraging words from former bodybuilder turned actor and then politician Arnold Schwarzenegger: "Strength does not come from winning. Your struggles develop your strengths. When you go through the hardships and decide not to surrender, that is strength" (Schwarzenegger, n.d).

Let's dive into the workouts! There is a detailed guide accompanying each workout advising you on how to complete it safely. The more challenging workouts include variations to cater to different fitness levels. There are also details of which muscle group is targeted and common pitfalls to avoid.

Wall Push-Ups

Muscle Groups Targeted

Shoulder (deltoids), triceps and chest muscles (pectoralis major and minor), back muscles (trapezius, rhomboids, and spinal stabilizers), and core muscles.

Instructions

1. Begin by standing with your legs shoulder-width apart and an arm's length away from the wall.
2. Place your hands on the wall at shoulder level, keeping them shoulder-width apart. If you feel like your arms are overstretched, stand slightly closer to the wall until you feel more comfortable.
3. Lean your body forward in a straight line, bending your elbows, until your forehead almost touches the wall. Keep your arms as close to your body as possible, rather than pushing them outward as you bend your elbows.
4. Straighten your arms as you move your body back to the starting position, completing one repetition (rep).
5. Complete 10 reps of the exercise.

Make It Easier

- Step closer to the wall, and have your arms wider apart.

Challenge Yourself

- Bring your hands closer together on the wall. You will feel the stretch in your upper arms and back.

- Step further away from the wall.

- Perform the exercise with one leg lifted, and alternate legs after 10 reps. If you try this variation, begin with a split stance (one foot in front of the other, as if you were about to start running a race).

Common Pitfalls

You may notice a tendency to want to arch your back or move your hips forward. Keep your back straight, and imagine a straight line from your head to your feet.

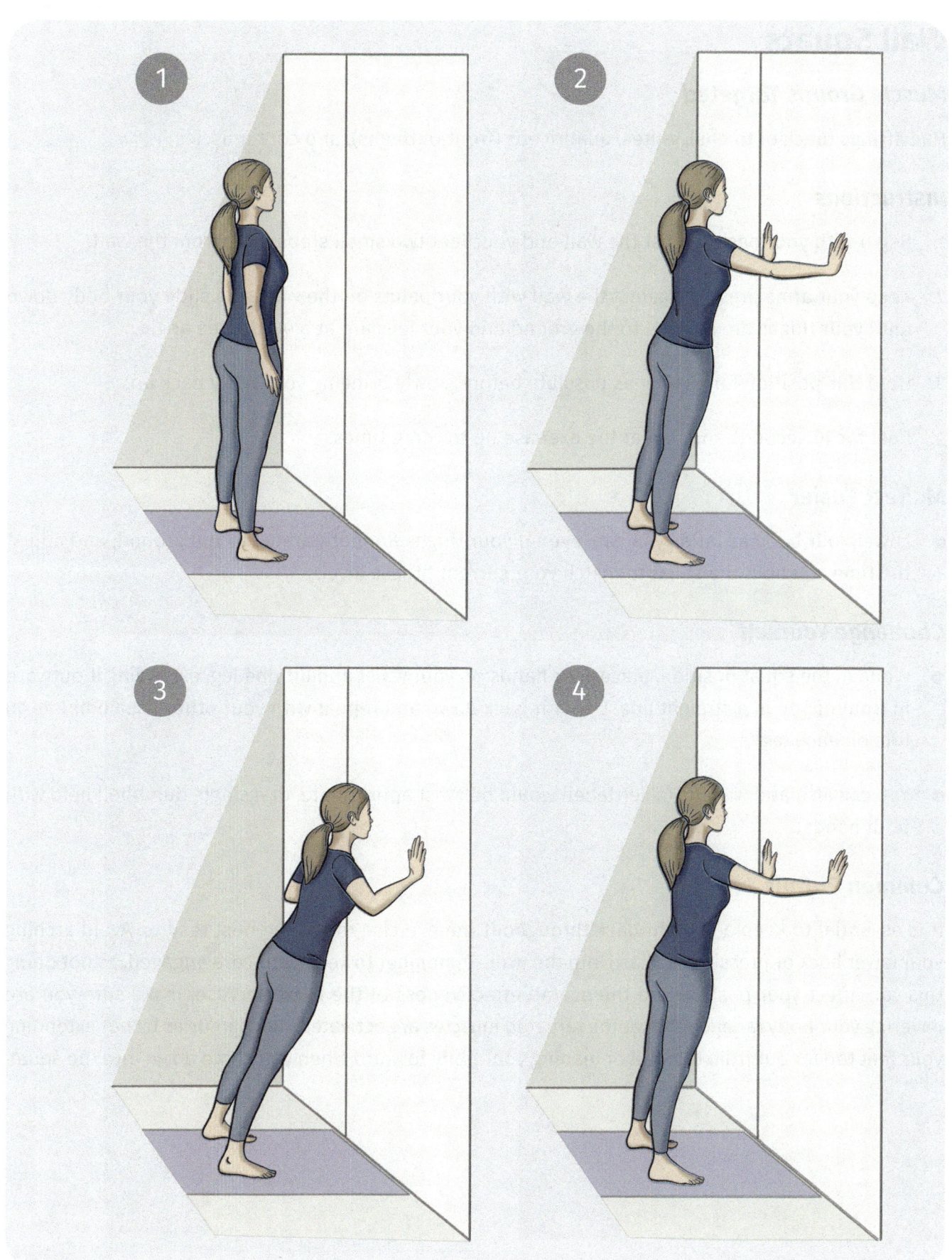

WALL PILATES WORKOUTS FOR WOMEN | 23

Wall Squats

Muscle Groups Targeted

Hamstrings (back of thighs), glutes, quadriceps (front of thighs), and core muscles.

Instructions

1. Begin with your back against the wall and your feet two small steps away from the wall.

2. Keep your arms pressed against the wall with your palms on the wall, and slide your body down until your thighs are parallel to the ground and your legs are at a 90-degree angle.

3. Hold this position for as long as possible before slowly bringing your body back up.

4. Rest for 10 seconds and repeat the exercise up to three times.

Make It Easier

- Lower your body as far as you can, even if your thighs are not parallel to the ground, and adjust the time you hold the squat to match your current fitness level.

Challenge Yourself

- While in the squat position, place your hands on your waist and lift one leg, extending it outward in front of you in a straight line. Lower it back down and repeat with your other leg. Complete 10 lifts on each leg.

- You can also add weights (a kettlebell would be most appropriate, or a single dumbbell held with both hands).

Common Pitfalls

It is essential to keep a straight back throughout the exercise to get the best results. Avoid arching your lower back or pressing too hard into the wall. Remember to keep your core engaged, as not doing this can affect your posture and the overall effectiveness of the exercise. Also, make sure you are lowering your body far enough that the targeted muscles are activated. Avoid injuries by not extending your feet too far out from the wall or leaning your body forward when you come down into the squat.

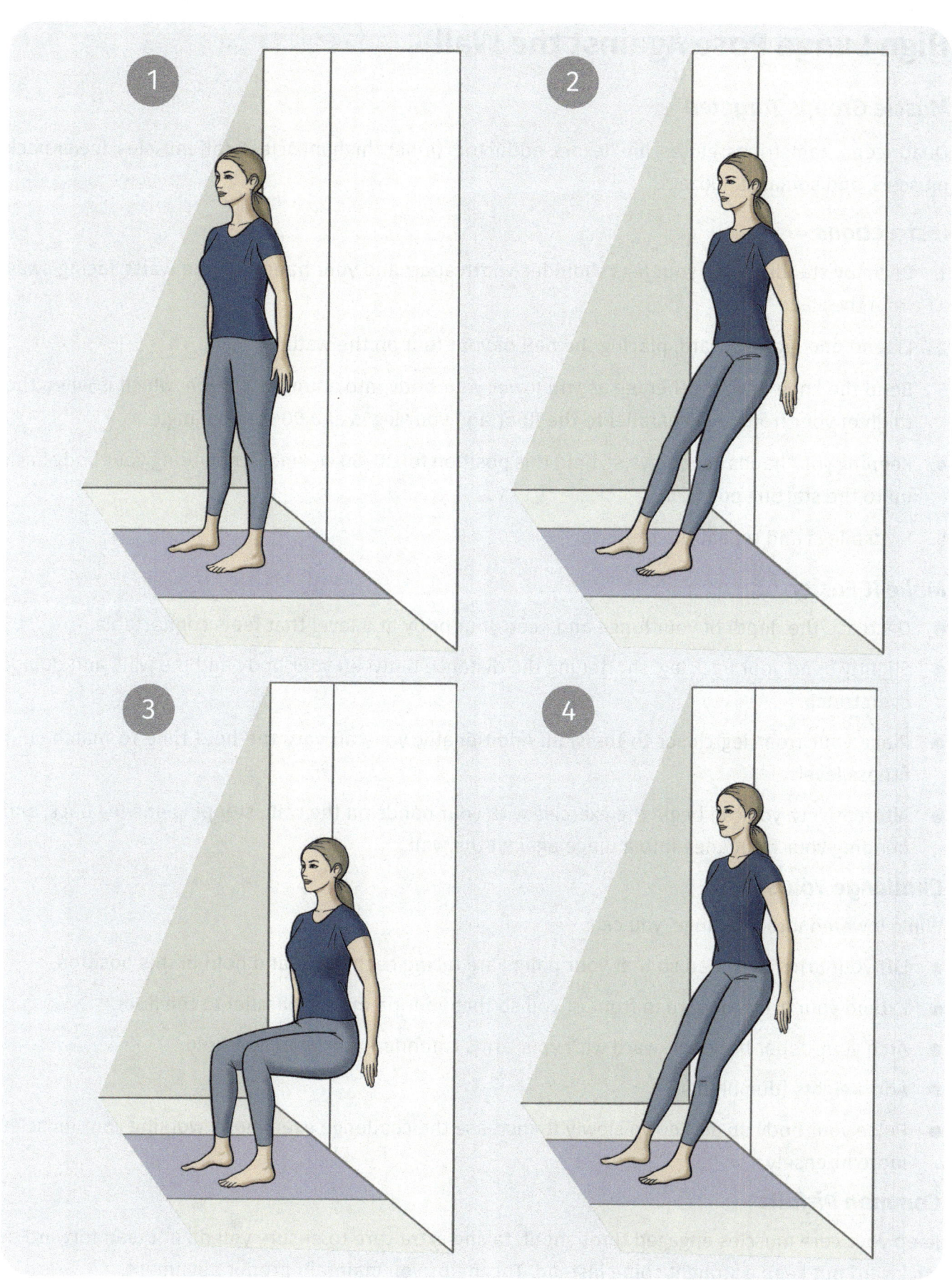

High Lunge Pose Against the Wall

Muscle Groups Targeted

Quadriceps, hamstrings, glutes, hip flexors, adductors (inner thigh muscles), calf muscles, lower back muscles, and spinal stabilizers.

Instructions

1. Begin by standing with your legs shoulder-width apart and your hands at your waist, facing away from the wall.
2. Extend one leg backward, placing the ball of your foot on the wall.
3. Bend the knee of your other leg as you lower your body into a lunge position, which is when the thigh of your front leg is parallel to the floor and your leg is at a 90-degree angle.
4. Keeping your hands at your waist, hold this position for 30–60 seconds, then bring your body back up to the starting position.
5. Switch legs and repeat the exercise.

Make It Easier

- Decrease the depth of your lunge and keep your body at a level that feels comfortable.
- Slightly bend your back leg, shortening the distance between your body and the wall, and do not overstretch.
- Place your front leg closer to the wall. Additionally, you can vary the hold time to match your fitness level.
- Alternatively, you can begin the exercise with your hands on the wall, stepping one leg back, and bending your front knee into a lunge against the wall.

Challenge Yourself

While lowered into the lunge, you can:

- Lift your arms overhead so that your palms are facing each other and hold in this position.
- Extend your arms forward in front of you so that your palms are parallel to the floor.
- Arch your upper back backward with your arms extended overhead and hold.
- Add weights (dumbbells).
- Pulse your body up and down slowly to increase the challenge even more, working your muscles more intensely.

Common Pitfalls

Keep your core muscles engaged throughout, taking extra care to ensure you do not lean forward or backward but keep a straight spine instead. This helps you maintain proper alignment.

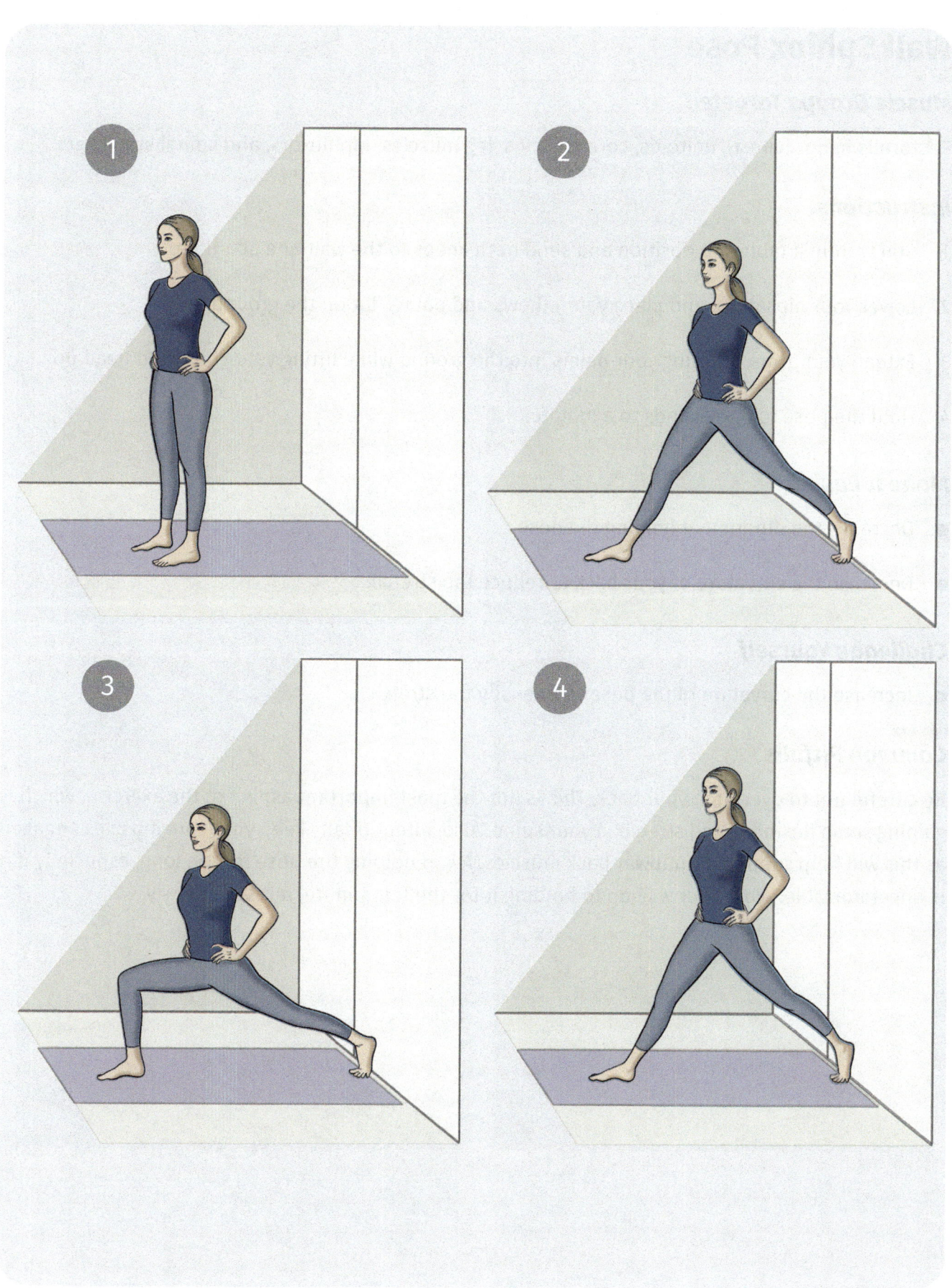

Wall Sphinx Pose

Muscle Groups Targeted

Pectoralis major (chest), deltoids, core muscles, leg muscles, hip flexors, and spinal stabilizers.

Instructions

1. Start out in a table-top position and send both knees to the wall one at a time.

2. Lower your hips down and place your elbows and palms flat on the ground.

3. Extend your arms, pressing your palms into the ground while lifting your chest and head up.

4. Hold the pose for 15 seconds to a minute.

Make It Easier

- Decrease the duration of holding the pose.
- Decrease the curvature of your back to reduce the stretch.

Challenge Yourself

- Increase the curvature of the pose to intensify the stretch.

Common Pitfalls

Be careful not to over-arch your back. This is not the most important aspect of the exercise, which is gaining some flexibility and stretch in your spine. Also, intentionally keep your core muscles engaged as this will help support your lower back muscles. Avoid holding the pose for too long, especially if it is uncomfortable. Work your way up to holding it for the full minute, but start slowly.

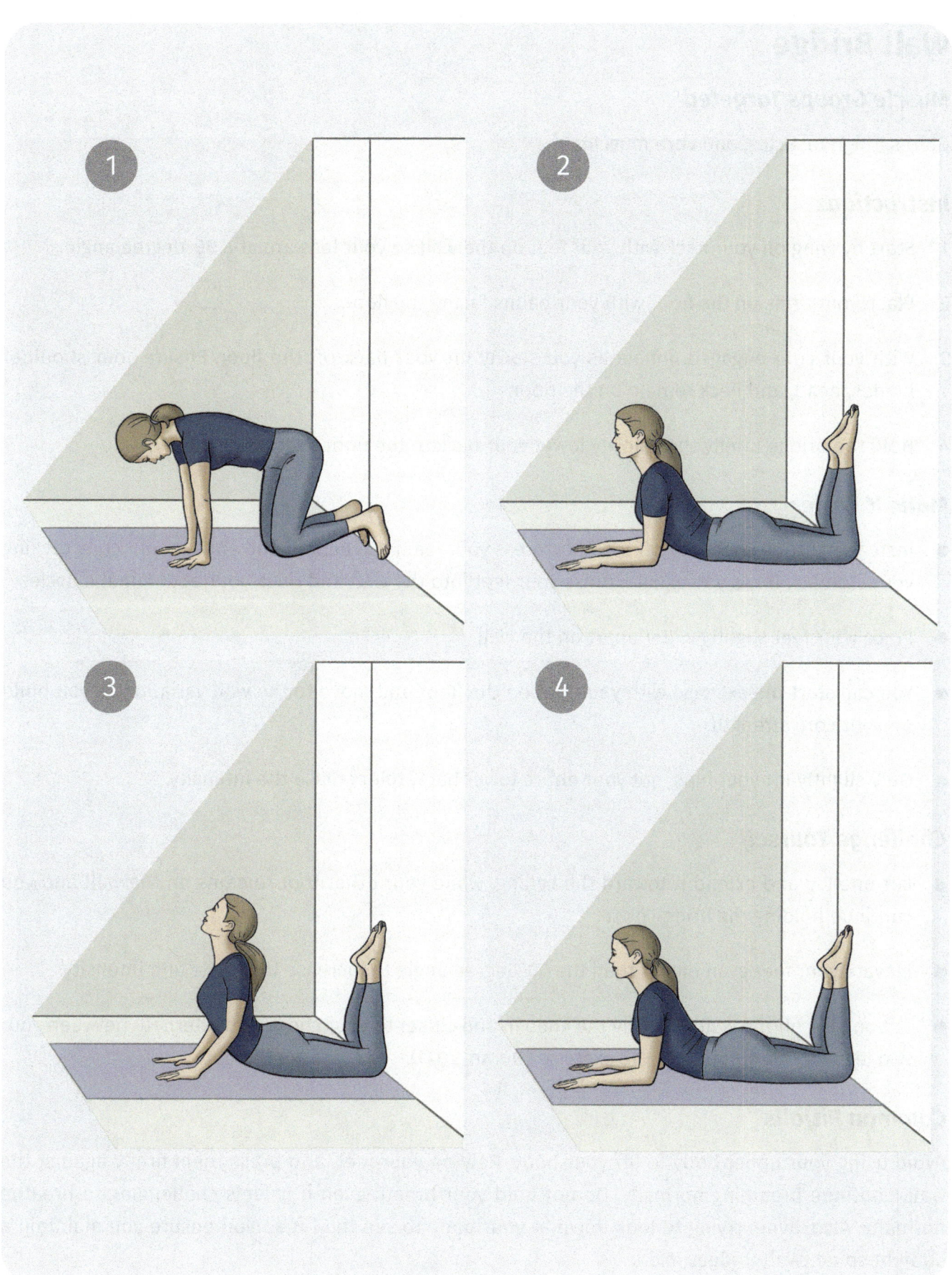

WALL PILATES WORKOUTS FOR WOMEN | 29

Wall Bridge

Muscle Groups Targeted

Glutes, thigh muscles, and core muscles.

Instructions

1. Start by lying on your back with your feet on the wall so your legs are at a 90-degree angle.

2. Place your arms on the floor with your palms facing the floor.

3. With your core engaged, inhale as you slowly lift your back off the floor. Ensure your shoulder blades, head, and neck remain on the floor.

4. Hold the bridge briefly then slowly lower your back to the floor again (Daisy, 2021).

Make It Easier

- Instead of lifting your back off the floor, press your feet into the wall and engage your core, tucking your stomach in. As you exhale, press your feet into the wall and relax your abdominal muscles.

- Place your feet slightly wider apart on the wall.

- You can start the exercise with your feet on the floor and move to the wall variation as you build up your core strength.

- Only slightly lift your hips, not your entire lower back, to decrease the intensity.

Challenge Yourself

- Lift one leg and extend it toward the ceiling, while your other foot remains on the wall and you continue holding the bridge pose.

- Elevate your feet even higher than the 90-degree angle to increase the angle and intensity.

- Lift one leg off the wall, bringing the knee in and closer to your chest, and alternate between your two legs for the duration of the exercise (Quinn, 2021).

Common Pitfalls

Avoid using your upper body to lift your body. Rely on your feet, and press them firmly against the wall. Continue breathing normally. Do not hold your breath even if it feels challenging to breathe normally. Also, avoid trying to look down at your body to see the lift so you ensure you maintain a straight spine (Wall Bridges, n.d.).

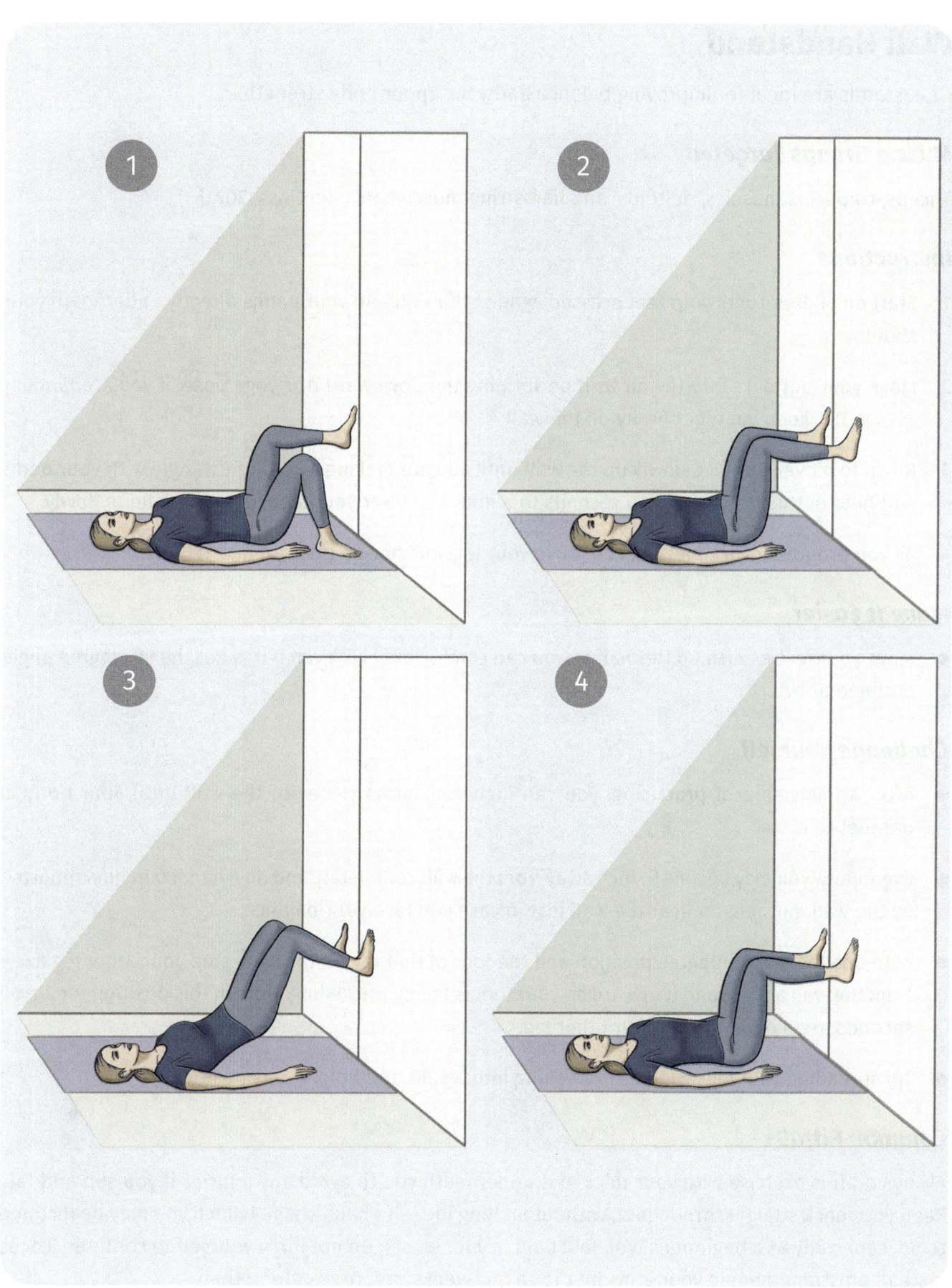

Wall Handstand

Handstands are ideal for improving balance and your upper body strength.

Muscle Groups Targeted

Triceps, trapezius muscles, deltoids, and hamstring muscles (MasterClass, 2021).

Instructions

1. Start on all fours with your feet pressed against the wall and your palms directly underneath your shoulders.

2. Move your buttocks into the air as if performing the downward dog yoga pose, if you are familiar with it. But keep your feet firmly on the wall.

3. Begin to move your feet slowly up the wall until you are making a 90-degree angle with your body, and hold in this position for 20 seconds to a minute. Lower your legs back to the floor slowly.

4. As you progress over time, you can move your legs further up the wall (Morris, 2023).

Make It Easier

- Move your feet as high up the wall as you can comfortably go, even if it is not the 90-degree angle outlined above.

Challenge Yourself

- After a few weeks of practicing, you can inch your arms closer to the wall until your body is parallel to it.

- Eventually, you may be able to inch away from the wall completely and do a handstand unsupported by the wall, but remain near the wall just in case you lose your balance.

- With one leg in a 90-degree position and the foot of that leg on the wall, step your other leg away from the wall and extend it upward so your foot is facing the ceiling. Hold in this position for 20–60 seconds, then repeat using your other leg.

- Try spreading your legs wide as if breaking into a split and hold in this position.

Common Pitfalls

Always do this exercise with your thick mat underneath you to avoid any injuries if you slip and fall. Keep your back straight throughout, without arching into a banana shape (which you may be inclined to do, especially as a beginner. If you feel pain in your wrists, do not force yourself to continue. Focus instead on strengthening your arms first for a few weeks before re-attempting.

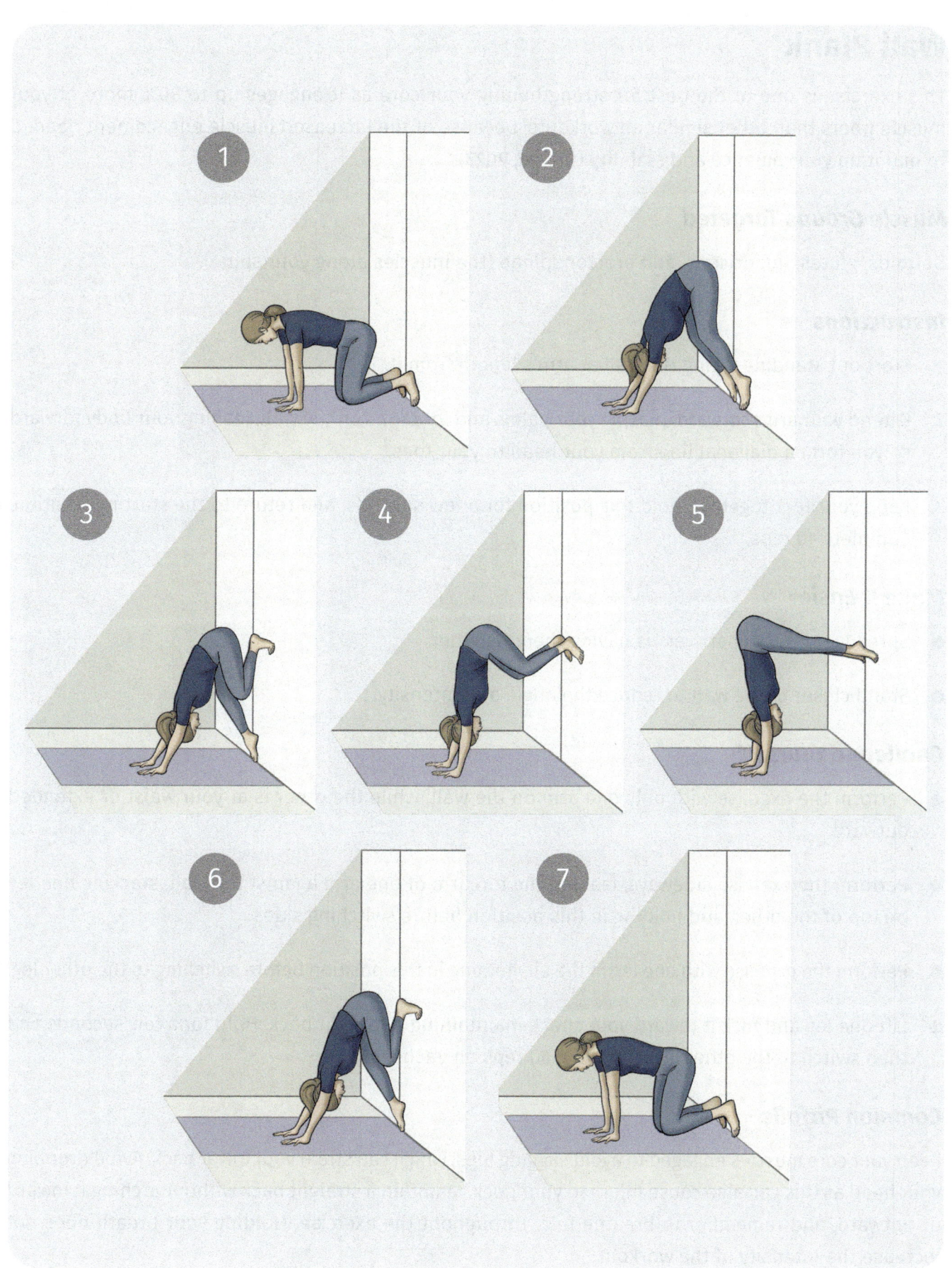

Wall Plank

This exercise is one of the best for strengthening your core as it engages up to 80% more of your muscle fibers than other similar ab workouts, because of the increased muscle engagement needed to maintain your balance and stability (Gracia, 2023).

Muscle Groups Targeted

Deltoids, glutes, quadriceps, and erector spinae (the muscles along your spine).

Instructions

1. Start out standing facing the wall at arm's length from it.

2. Extend your arms forward, placing your palms and forearms on the wall, leaning your body forward so you form a diagonal line from your head to your toes.

3. Keep your feet together, hold this position for a few seconds, and return to the starting position. Complete 10 reps.

Make It Easier

- Spread your feet apart versus having them together.

- Stand closer to the wall to reduce the angle and intensity.

Challenge Yourself

- Perform the exercise with only one arm on the wall, while the other is at your waist or extended outward.

- Perform the exercise sideways, leaning the forearm of one arm against the wall, stacking one leg on top of the other, and holding in this position before switching sides.

- Perform the exercise with one leg in the air, holding in this position before switching to the other leg.

- Lift one leg and tuck it toward your chest, maintaining a straight back. Hold for a few seconds and then switch to the other leg. Complete 10 reps on each leg.

Common Pitfalls

Keep your core muscles engaged to avoid sagging hips, which can strain your lower back. Avoid dropping your head as this can also cause injury to your neck. Maintain a straight back without arching it inward or outward, and remember to breathe fully throughout the exercise. Holding your breath does not increase the intensity of the workout.

Conclusion

Building your strength will be beneficial for the rest of the exercises in this guide, so I suggest you take your time here and work through the more difficult progressions as you strengthen not only the core powerhouse but your entire body. This is one of the reasons wall Pilates is so effective and uniquely positioned as a true full-body workout.

In the next chapter, we will get your heart rate going with exercises to improve your stamina.

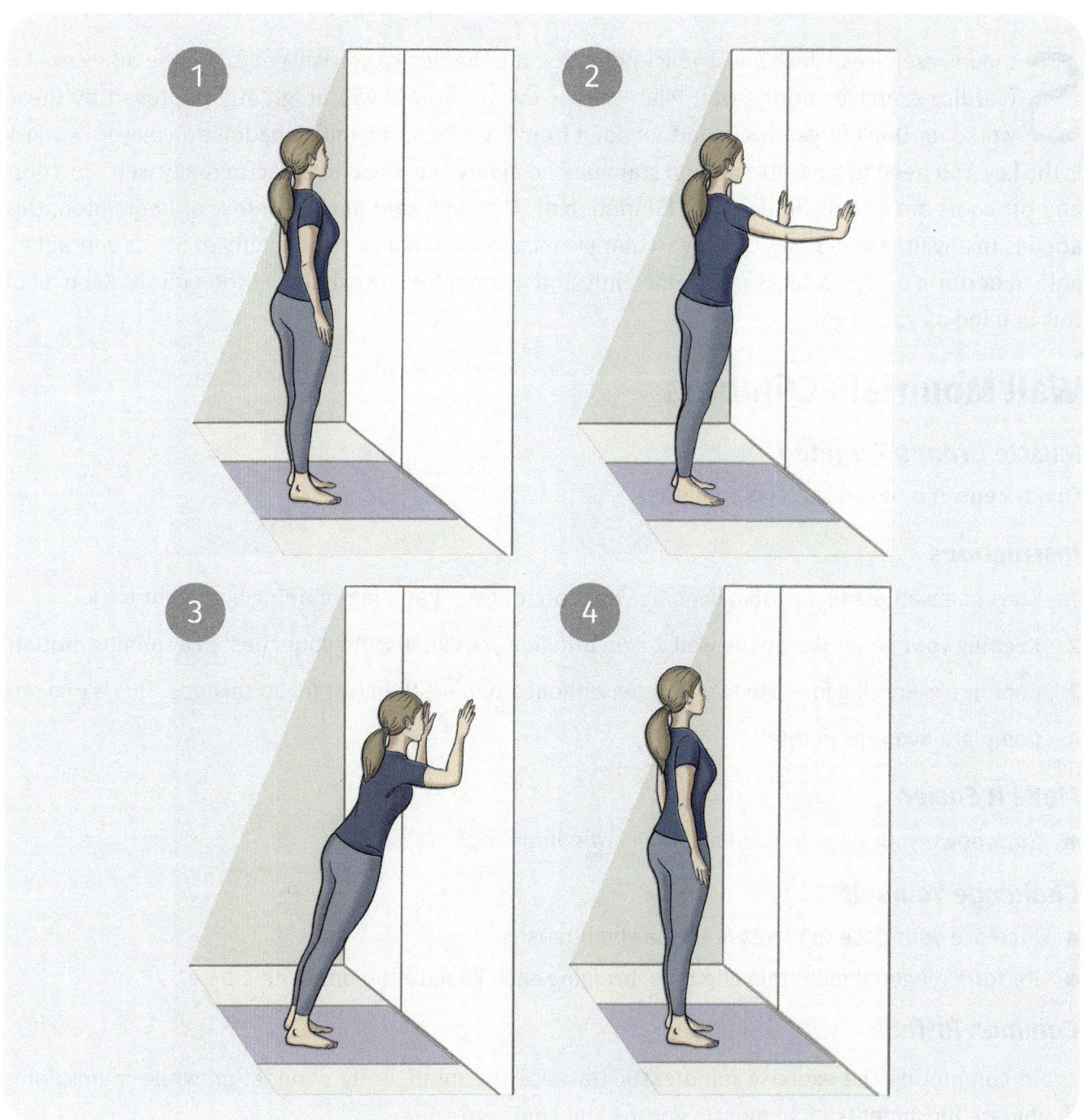

CHAPTER 5
BOOSTING STAMINA WITH WALL WORKOUTS

Stamina exercises, which boost your endurance, are the closest you will get to doing cardiovascular (cardio) exercises during wall Pilates. Your overall fitness will be greatly improved by these workouts. Don't forget this important point from P. V. Sindhu, an Indian badminton player: "Fitness is the key. You need to have strokes and stamina and agility; you need to exercise really well. On-court and off-court are equally important," (Sindhu, n.d). Although said in the context of badminton, this applies to any fitness journey. Cardiovascular exercises will enhance your quality of life as you will be able to perform everyday tasks more efficiently and without feeling exhausted too quickly. Keep all of this in mind as you begin.

Wall Mountain Climbers

Muscle Groups Targeted
Quadriceps, hip flexors, and core muscles.

Instructions
1. Start in a wall plank position, keeping your core engaged and maintaining a straight back.
2. Keeping your palms flat on the wall, begin bringing your knees into your chest in a running motion.
3. Continue exercising for up to two minutes without stopping, then rest for 30 seconds. This is one rep.
4. Complete five reps in total.

Make It Easier
- Slow down your pace to decrease the cardio intensity.

Challenge Yourself
- Increase your pace to increase the cardio intensity.
- Perform diagonal mountain climbers, bringing each knee to the opposite elbow.

Common Pitfalls
Avoid completing the exercise mindlessly. Harness the mind–body connection while maintaining deliberate movements of all muscle groups involved.

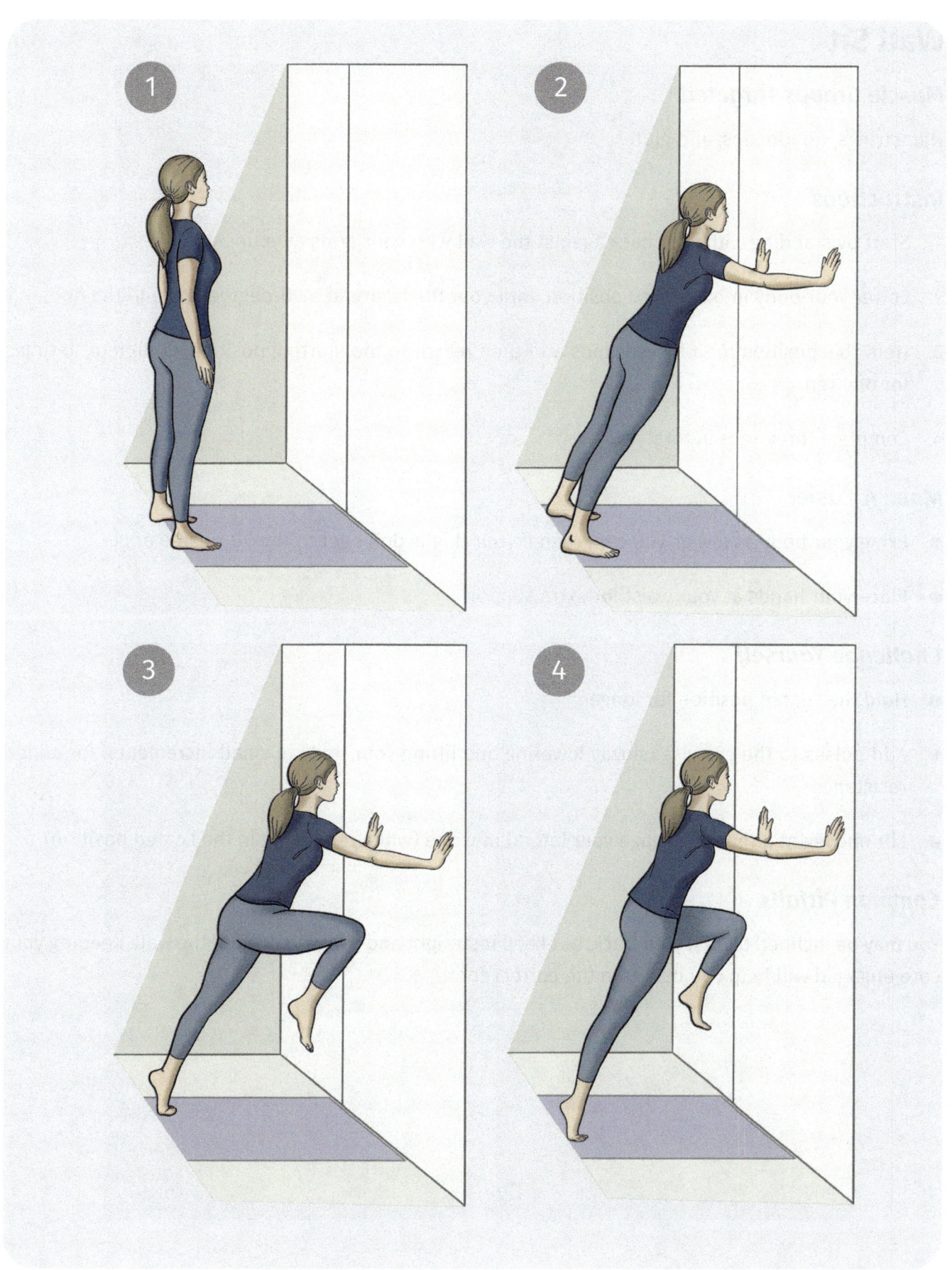

WALL PILATES WORKOUTS FOR WOMEN | 37

Wall Sit

Muscle Groups Targeted

Hamstrings, quadriceps, and glutes.

Instructions

1. Start by standing with your back against the wall with your arms at your sides.

2. Lower your body into a seated position until your thighs are at a 90-degree angle to the floor.

3. Hold this position for a few seconds and then return to the starting position. Complete 10 times for one rep.

4. Complete three reps in total.

Make It Easier

- Bring your body as low as you can, even if your thighs don't get to the 90-degree angle.

- Place your hands at your waist for extra support.

Challenge Yourself

- Hold the seated position for longer.

- Add pulses to the exercise (slowly lowering and lifting your body in small increments) for added resistance.

- Lift one leg at a time to engage your lateral muscles (while remaining in the seated position).

Common Pitfalls

You may be inclined to arch your back, but keep it straight and pressed against the wall. Keeping your core engaged will help you maintain the correct form.

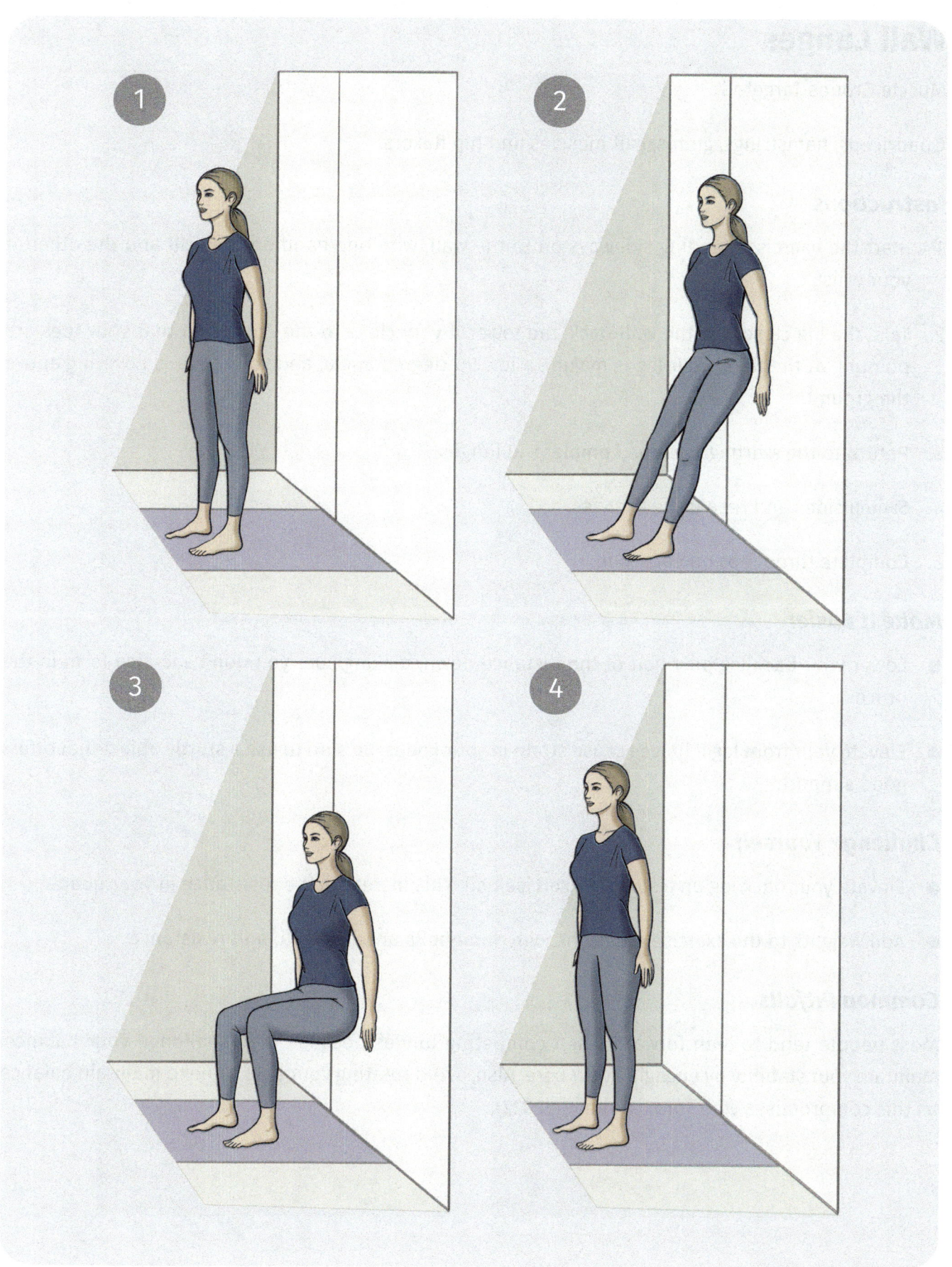

WALL PILATES WORKOUTS FOR WOMEN | 39

Wall Lunges

Muscle Groups Targeted

Quadriceps, hamstrings, glutes, calf muscles and hip flexors.

Instructions

1. Start the exercise standing sideways on to the wall, with one hand on the wall and the other at your waist.

2. Take the leg closest to the wall back and lower it very close to the ground so that your toes are pointing at the floor, your leg is making a low 90-degree angle, and your knee is hovering above the ground.

3. Return to the starting position Complete 10 lunges.

4. Switch sides and repeat the exercise.

5. Complete three reps on each side.

Make It Easier

- Lower your back leg only half of the distance down, making sure you don't sacrifice form in the process.

- Elevate your front leg if lunges cause strain in your knees. Be sure to use a sturdy object that offers good support.

Challenge Yourself

- Elevate your back leg on a stool or exercise ball. This increases the resistance in your quads.

- Add weights to the exercise either through dumbbells or barbells to add resistance.

Common Pitfalls

Most people tend to lean forward when competing lunges because they challenge your balance. Maintain your stability by engaging your core. Also, avoid rotating your back knee to maintain balance as this compromises your form (Waehner, 2022).

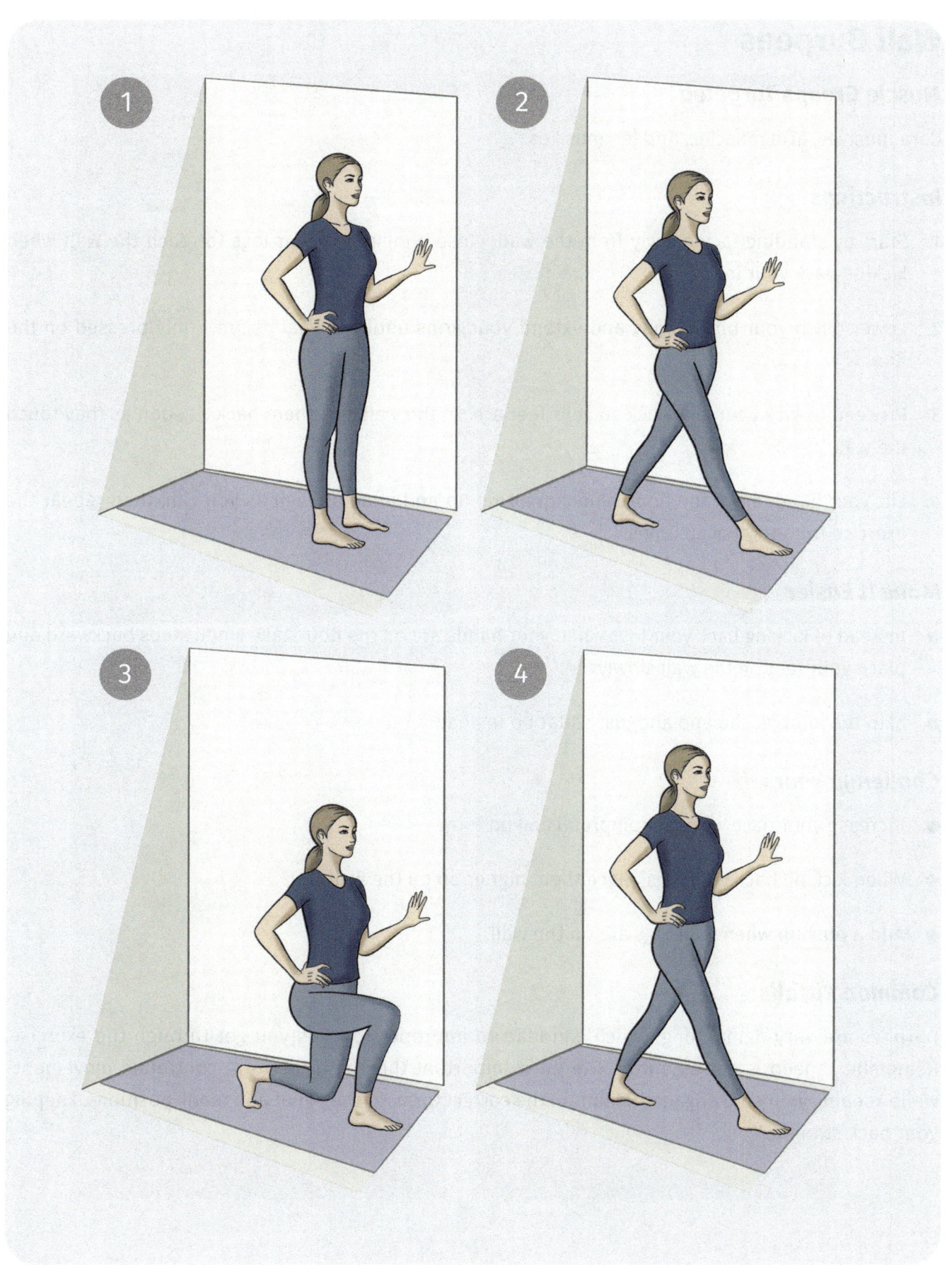

Wall Burpees

Muscle Groups Targeted

Core muscles, arm muscles, and leg muscles.

Instructions

1. Start by standing facing away from the wall, close enough for your legs to reach the wall when kicking back your legs.

2. Lower down your upper body and extend your arms until your palms are firmly pressed on the floor.

3. Proceed to kick your legs back so your feet are on the wall kick them back as soon as they touch the wall.

4. Lift your hands from the floor while squatting up and jump as high as you can, then repeat the exercise for a total of 10 times.

Make It Easier

- Instead of kicking back your legs when your hands are on the floor, take small steps backward and place your feet on the wall slowly.

- Skip the jump at the end and just squat up instead.

Challenge Yourself

- Increase your pace without compromising on form.

- When kicking back your legs, place them higher up on the wall.

- Add a pushup when your legs are on the wall.

Common Pitfalls

Burpees are very demanding, which can lead to improper form as you get through the exercise. Remember, speed is not essential. The most important thing is to perform controlled movements while keeping your core engaged. Maintain the correct form for the squat and plank positions, keeping your back straight.

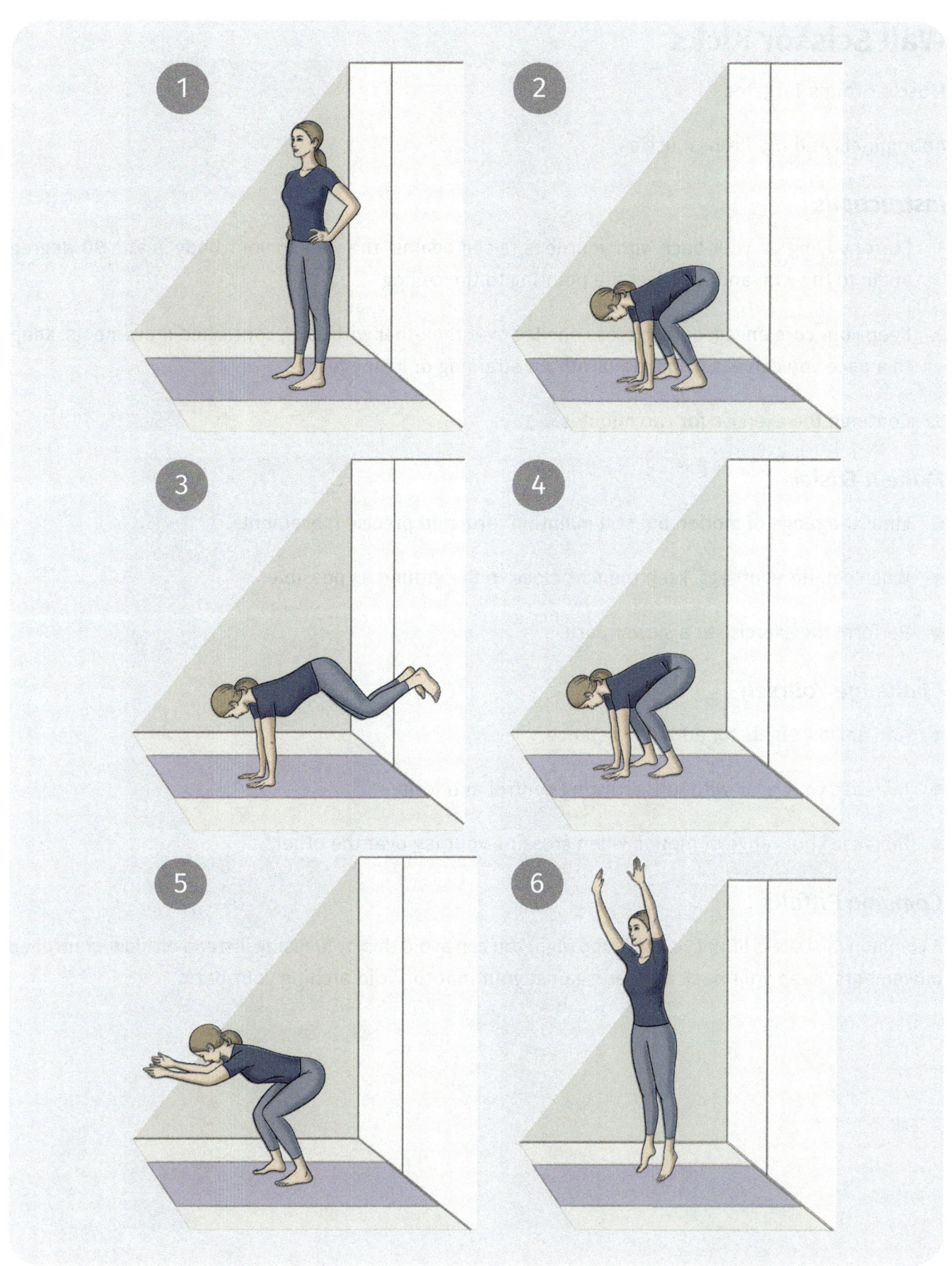

Wall Scissor Kicks

Muscle Groups Targeted

Abdominals and hip flexor muscles.

Instructions

1. Start by lying on your back with your legs raised against the wall so your body is at a 90-degree angle to the wall and your feet are pointing to the ceiling.

2. Keep your core engaged, then cross one leg over the other with slow, controlled movements. Keep to a pace you can easily maintain without straining or losing form.

3. Continue the exercise for two minutes.

Make It Easier

- Limit the range of motion but still maintain form and precise movements.
- When you lift your legs, keep them as close to the ground as possible.
- Perform the exercise at a slower pace.

Challenge Yourself

- Add ankle weights for added resistance.
- Increase your pace without sacrificing control and form.
- Increase your range of motion when crossing your leg over the other.

Common Pitfalls

A common mistake is lifting your legs too high. You can avoid this by focusing instead on slow, controlled movements. Keep your back pressed against your mat to avoid arching your back.

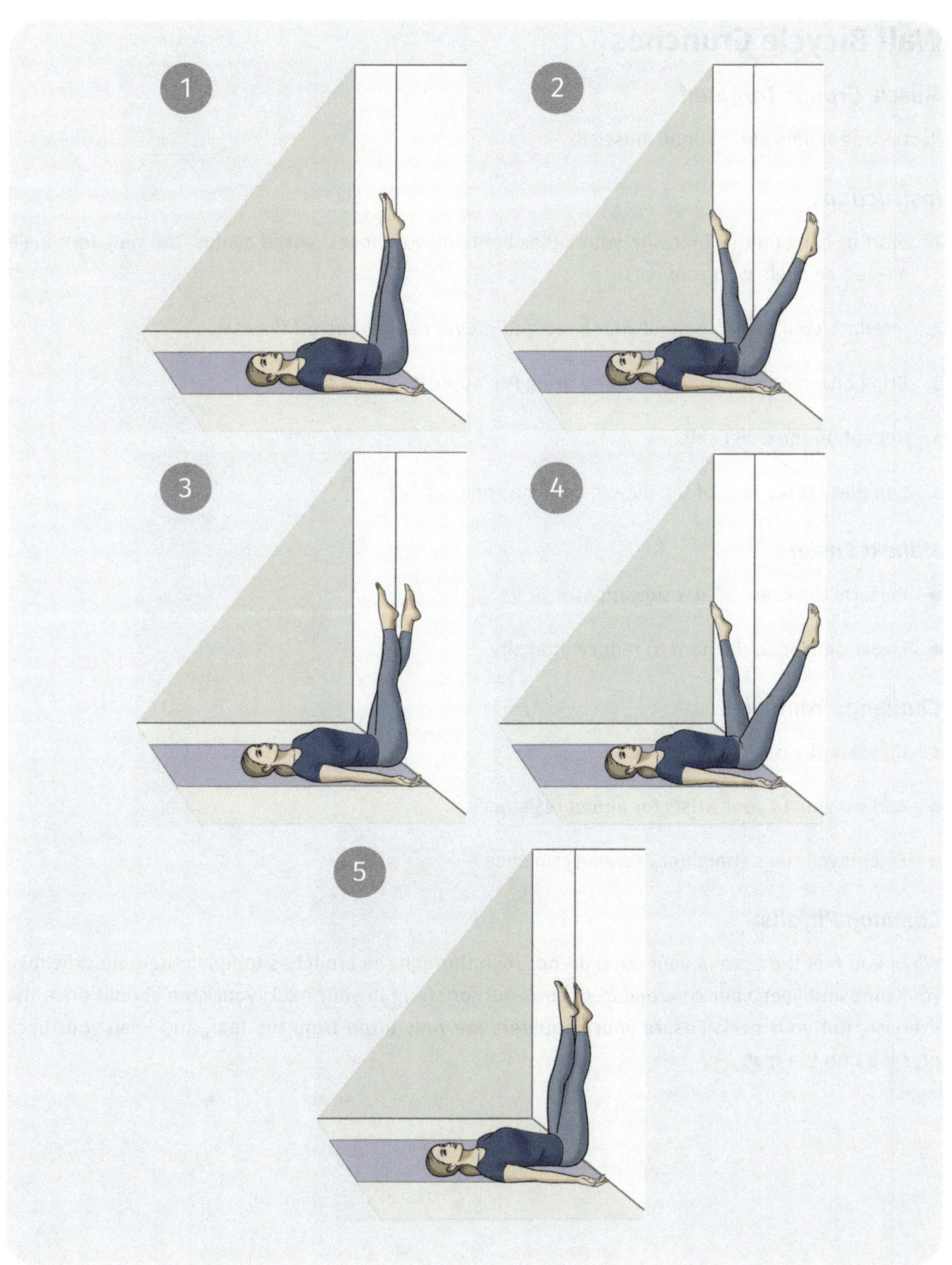

Wall Bicycle Crunches

Muscle Groups Targeted

Rectus abdominis and oblique muscles.

Instructions

1. Start by lying on the floor with your knees bent and your feet pressed against the wall, forming a 90-degree angle with your legs.

2. Interlace your fingers behind your head and lift your shoulders off the mat.

3. Bring one knee into your chest, and bring the opposite elbow toward it.

4. Repeat on the other side.

5. Complete three reps of ten bicycle crunches on each leg.

Make It Easier

- Perform the exercise at a slower pace.

- Lower one leg to the floor to reduce intensity.

Challenge Yourself

- Increase the pace of the exercise.

- Add weights to your wrists for added resistance.

- Extend your legs straighter between crunches.

Common Pitfalls

When you feel the burn in your core, do not rush through the crunches to finish them quickly. Take your time and keep your core engaged. Look out for strain in your neck; your core should drive the exercise, not your neck. Ensure your shoulders are fully lifted from the mat, and keep your back pressed into the mat.

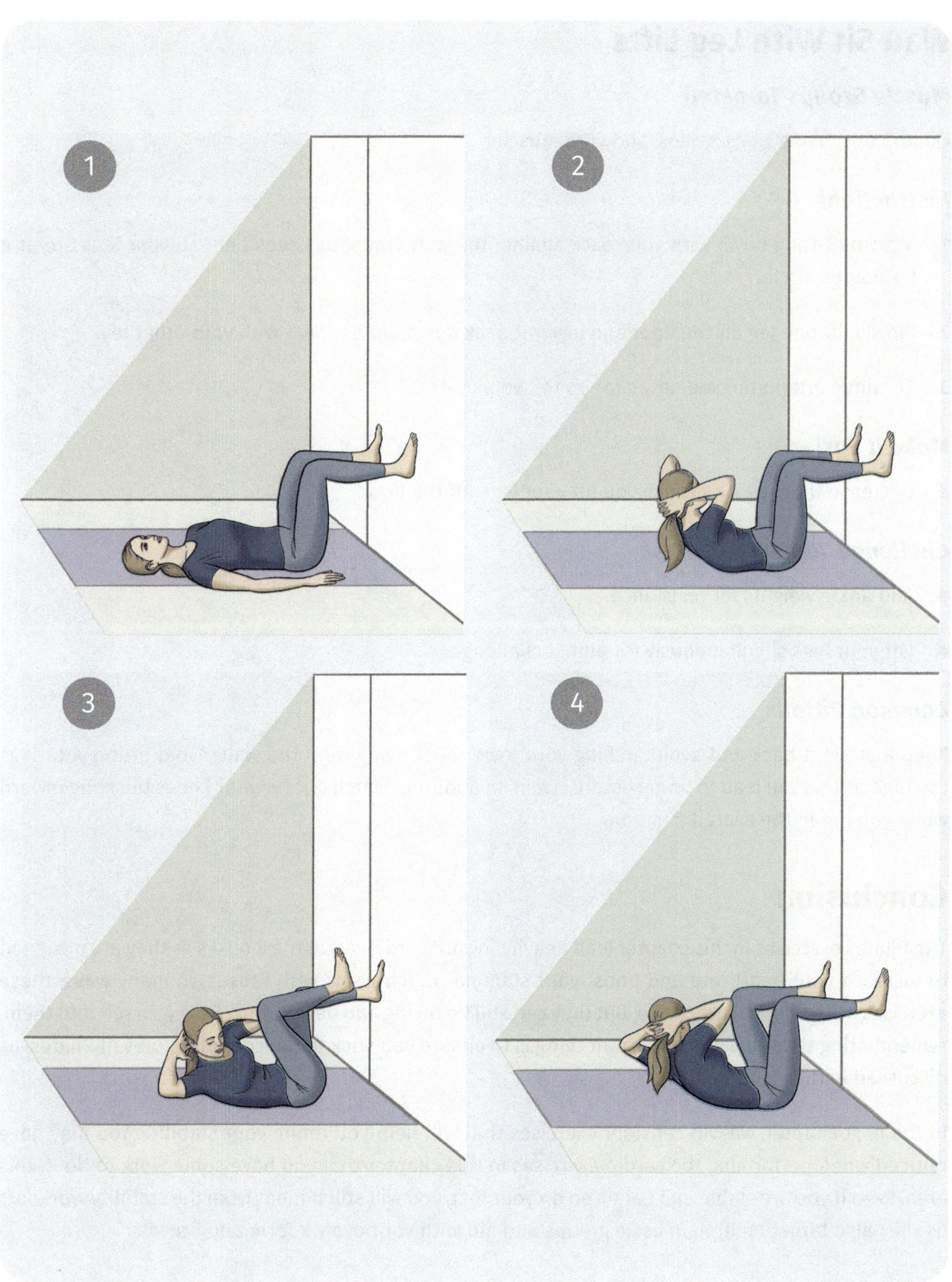

Wall Sit With Leg Lifts

Muscle Groups Targeted

Quadriceps, hamstrings, glutes, and core muscles.

Instructions

1. Start by sitting down with your back against the wall and your knees bent so your legs are at a 90-degree angle.

2. Slowly lift one leg off the floor and lower it back down, then repeat with your other leg.

3. Continue alternating leg raises for up to two minutes.

Make It Easier

- Decrease the height to which you lift your legs off the floor.

Challenge Yourself

- Add ankle weights for resistance.

- Lift your legs simultaneously for added challenge.

Common Pitfalls

Keep a straight back and avoid arching your lower back away from the wall. Avoid lifting your legs too high as this will lead to unnecessary strain. In addition, watch out for your knees buckling inward while you are in the seated position.

Conclusion

The Pilates exercises in this chapter lean heavily toward cardiovascular exercises as they are designed to increase your heart rate and boost your stamina, which helps with fitness. In many ways, these exercises are lower-impact cardio, but they can still be taxing and demanding. Ease yourself into them, remembering that the most important thing is to ensure you stick to the core principles of Pilates, as discussed earlier in the book.

In the next chapter, we will consider exercises that will help you refine your stability. You may have noticed when performing the cardio exercises in this chapter that you have some work to do in this area. Even if you are stable and balanced on your feet, you will still benefit from the stability workouts as they also target multiple muscle groups and aid with your overall form and fitness.

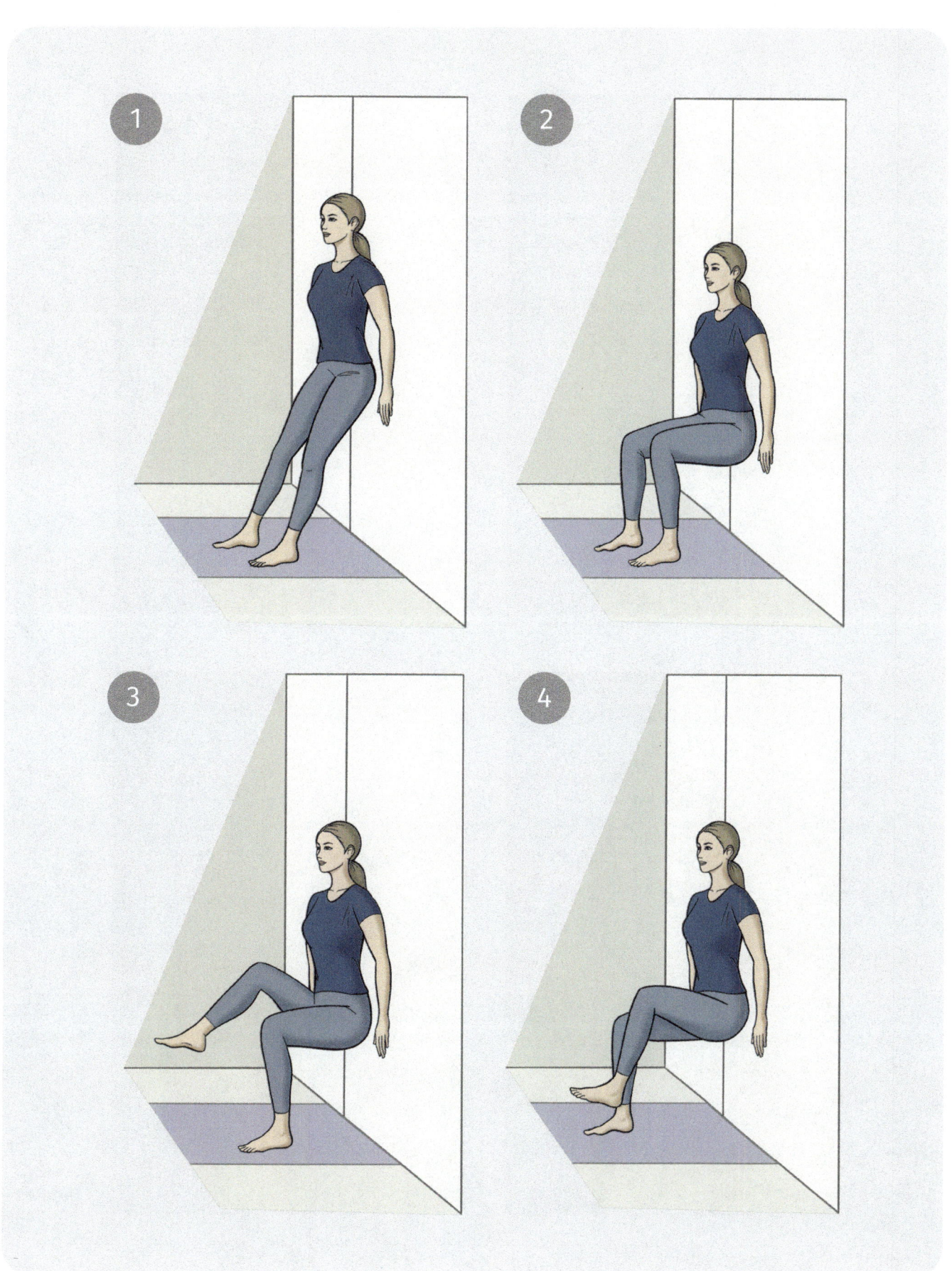

CHAPTER 6
ENHANCING STABILITY WITH WALL PILATES

By now, you appreciate the value of balance and stability in your ability to perform wall Pilates. If this has proven to be a weak area for you, you will love this chapter! The following exercises will help you improve your spinal mobility and posture even if you are fairly steady. We are halfway through the exercises, and you have done the hardest part, according to Erin Gray, an American actress: "The hardest thing about exercise is to start doing it. Once you are doing exercise regularly, the hardest thing to do is stop it," (Feiereisen & Milbrand, 2023).

I hope you are beginning to establish the habit so that by the time we reach the 30-day challenge, you are ready to go with full confidence that you will see it through. Let's begin!

Wall Angels

Muscle Groups Targeted

Upper and lower back muscles.

Instructions

1. Start by sitting with your back against the wall and your legs extended outward, forming an "L" shape with your body.
2. Extend your arms outward onto the wall with your elbows in line with your shoulders.
3. Slowly move your arms upward until they are extended over your head. Move your back and arm muscles with precision, keeping your back pressed into the wall.
4. Lower your arms back down with your upper arms parallel to the ground.
5. Repeat the exercise 10–15 times.

Make It Easier

You can lie on the floor instead, with your legs extended up the wall, and perform the exercise on the floor. This will be helpful if you have lower back or neck pain.

Practice the exercise one arm at a time to decrease the tension on your spine.

Challenge Yourself

- Engage your core while performing the exercise.
- Add light weights for added resistance.

Common Pitfalls

It is easy to assume this exercise is simple and can be rushed through, but this compromises its effectiveness. Take your time and make precise, controlled movements throughout. You should also pay attention to form, ensuring your back is pressed into the wall and your hips are sturdy. Avoid shifting or lifting your hips by ensuring you are firmly seated on the floor. Also, keep your neck tucked in to avoid leaning forward or straining your neck to reach overhead. Don't overstretch; start slowly and work up to reaching further as you become more flexible.

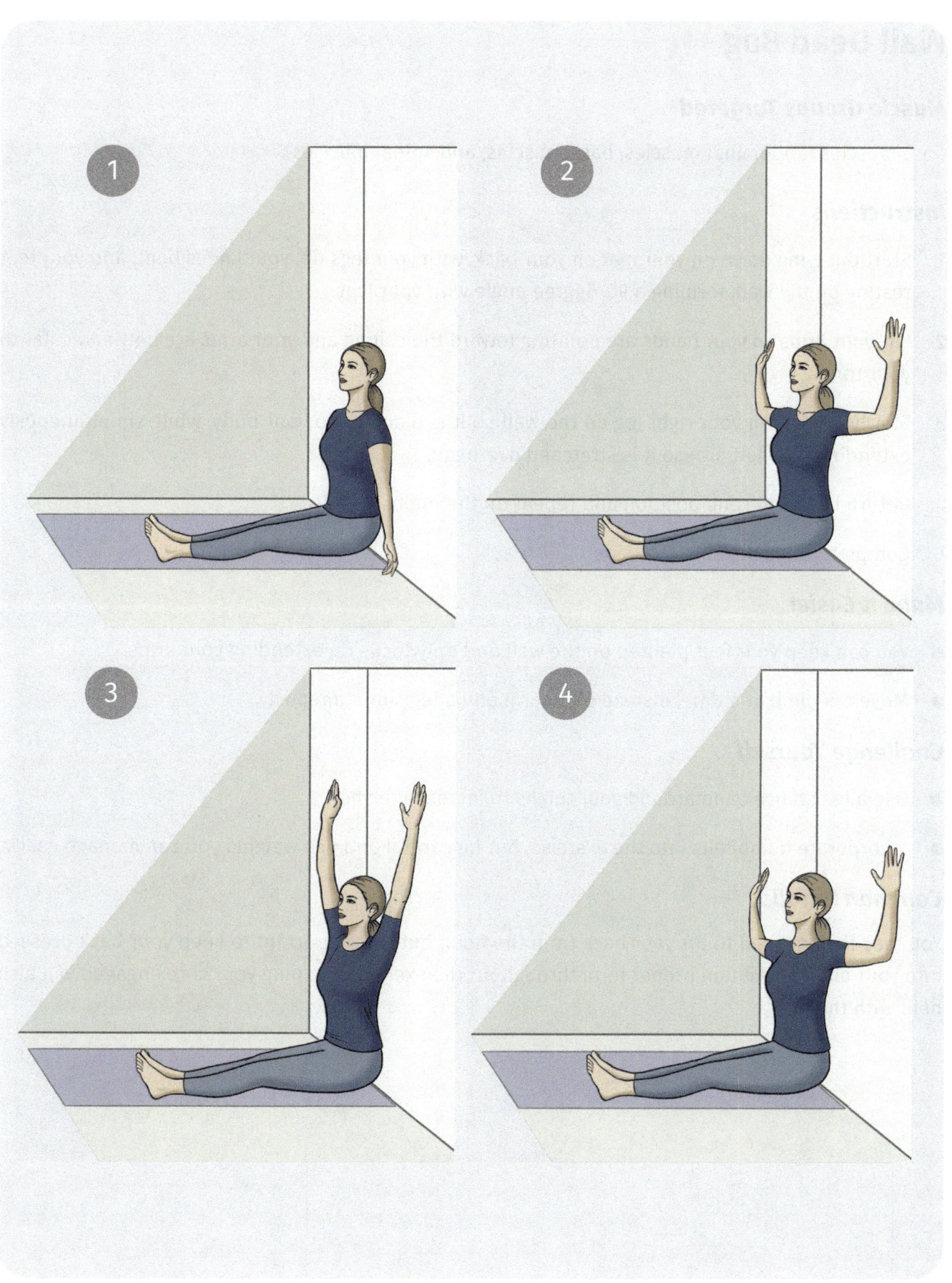

Wall Dead Bug

Muscle Groups Targeted

Core muscles (abdominal muscles, back muscles, and spinal muscles).

Instructions

1. Start out lying down on your mat on your back, with your legs up, your knees bent, and your feet resting on the wall, forming a 90-degree angle with your legs.
2. Lift your arms so your hands are pointing toward the ceiling and your arms are perpendicular to your torso.
3. Slowly straighten your right leg up the wall so it is diagonal to your body, while simultaneously extending your left arm so it is stretched overhead.
4. Return to the starting position and repeat on the opposite side.
5. Complete 10–15 reps on each side.

Make It Easier

- You can keep your feet planted on the wall and only focus on extending your arms.
- Move one limb at a time, instead of an arm and a leg simultaneously.

Challenge Yourself

- Use a resistance band around your thighs to increase tension.
- Incorporate dumbbells into the exercise, but be careful and use weights you can manage easily.

Common Pitfalls

You may feel inclined to lift your back from the floor, but it is important to keep your back pressed into your mat to maintain proper form throughout the exercise. Keeping your core engaged will also help with this.

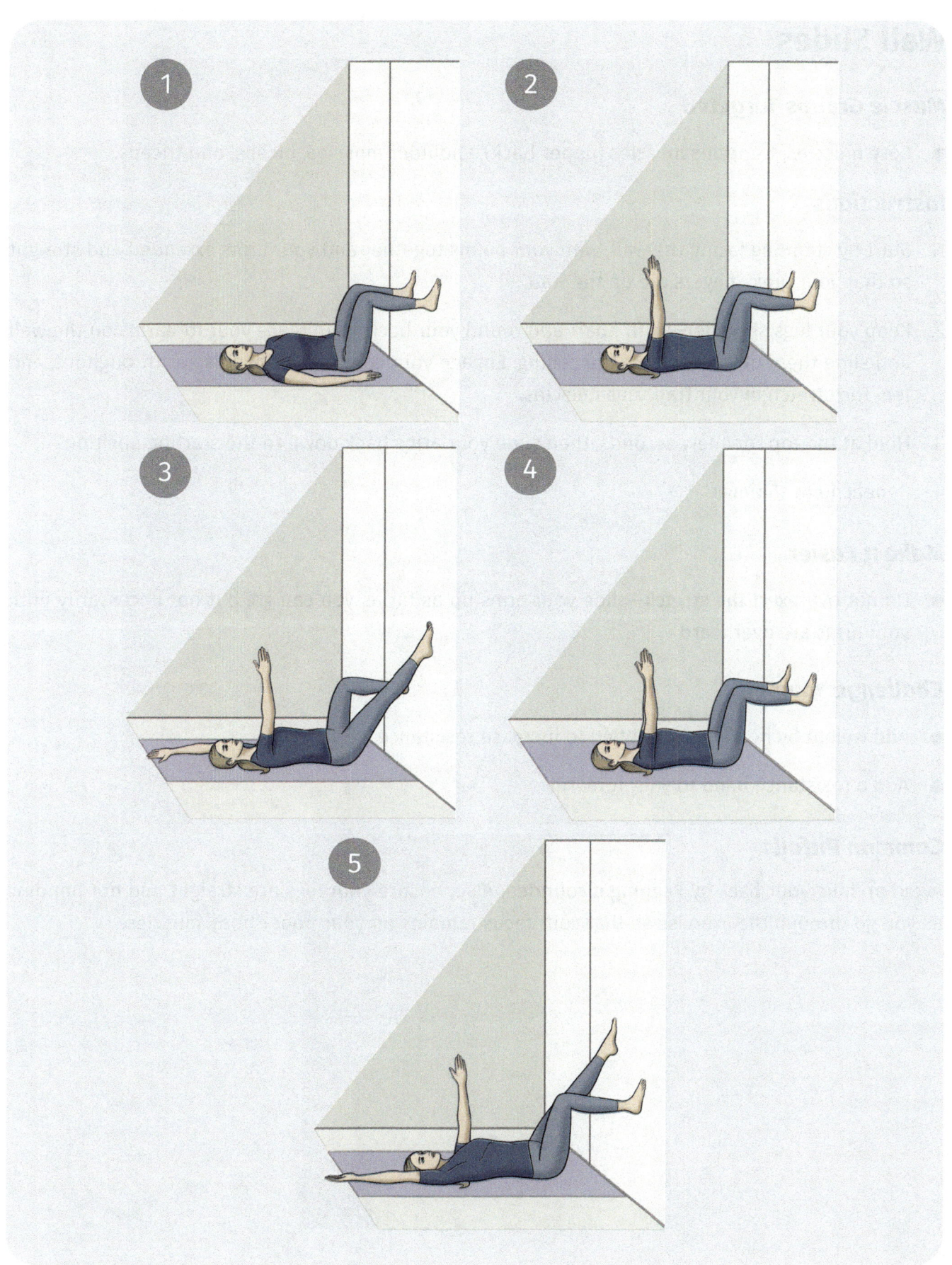

Wall Slides

Muscle Groups Targeted

- Core muscles, trapezius muscles (upper back), shoulder muscles, biceps, and triceps.

Instructions

1. Start by standing facing the wall, with your palms together and your arms extended and straight so that your pinky fingers are on the wall.

2. Keep your legs shoulder-width apart and round your back, then place your forearms on the wall and slide them upward toward the ceiling. Engage your core and back muscles throughout, and feel the stretch in your trapezius muscles.

3. Hold at the top for a few seconds, then slide your arms back down to the starting position.

4. Repeat 10 to 15 times.

Make It Easier

- Do not overexert the stretch—slide your arms up as far as you can go, but not necessarily until your arms are overheard.

Challenge Yourself

- Add weight by holding a dumbbell to increase resistance.
- Add a resistance band to your forearms.

Common Pitfalls

Avoid arching your back by keeping it rounded. Also, ensure your legs are straight and not bending as you go through the exercise so that your focus remains on your upper body muscles.

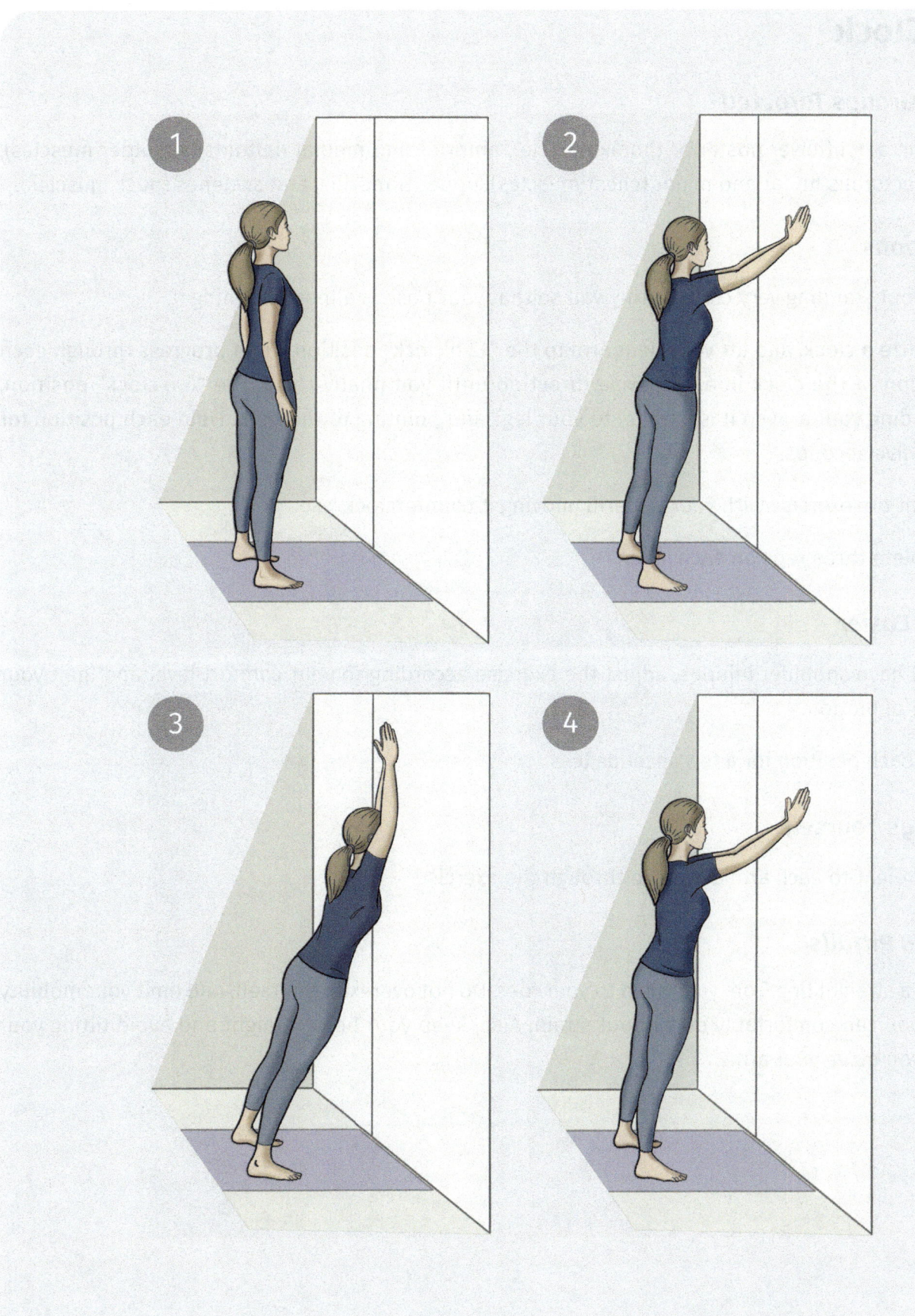

Wall Clock

Muscle Groups Targeted

Latissimus dorsi (lower posterior thorax muscle), anterior and medial deltoids (shoulder muscles), biceps, pectoralis minor and major (chest muscles), upper trapezius, and scalenes (neck muscles).

Instructions

1. Start out standing very close to the wall so that your nose is almost touching it.

2. Visualize a clock, and lift your right arm to the "12 o'clock" position. Then progress through each position of the clock in a clockwise direction until you finally reach the "6 o'clock" position, extending your arm so it is parallel to your legs and pointing to the floor. Hold each position for up to five seconds.

3. Repeat the exercise with your left arm, moving it counterclockwise.

4. Complete three reps on each side.

Make It Easier

- If you have shoulder injuries, adjust the exercise according to your comfort level and limit your range of motion.

- Hold each position for a few seconds less.

Challenge Yourself

- Add weight to each arm as you go through the exercise.

Common Pitfalls

Maintain a straight line from your head to your toes. Do not overexert yourself, and limit your mobility to what you can comfortably do without strain. Also, keep your head straight and avoid tilting your neck as you move your arms.

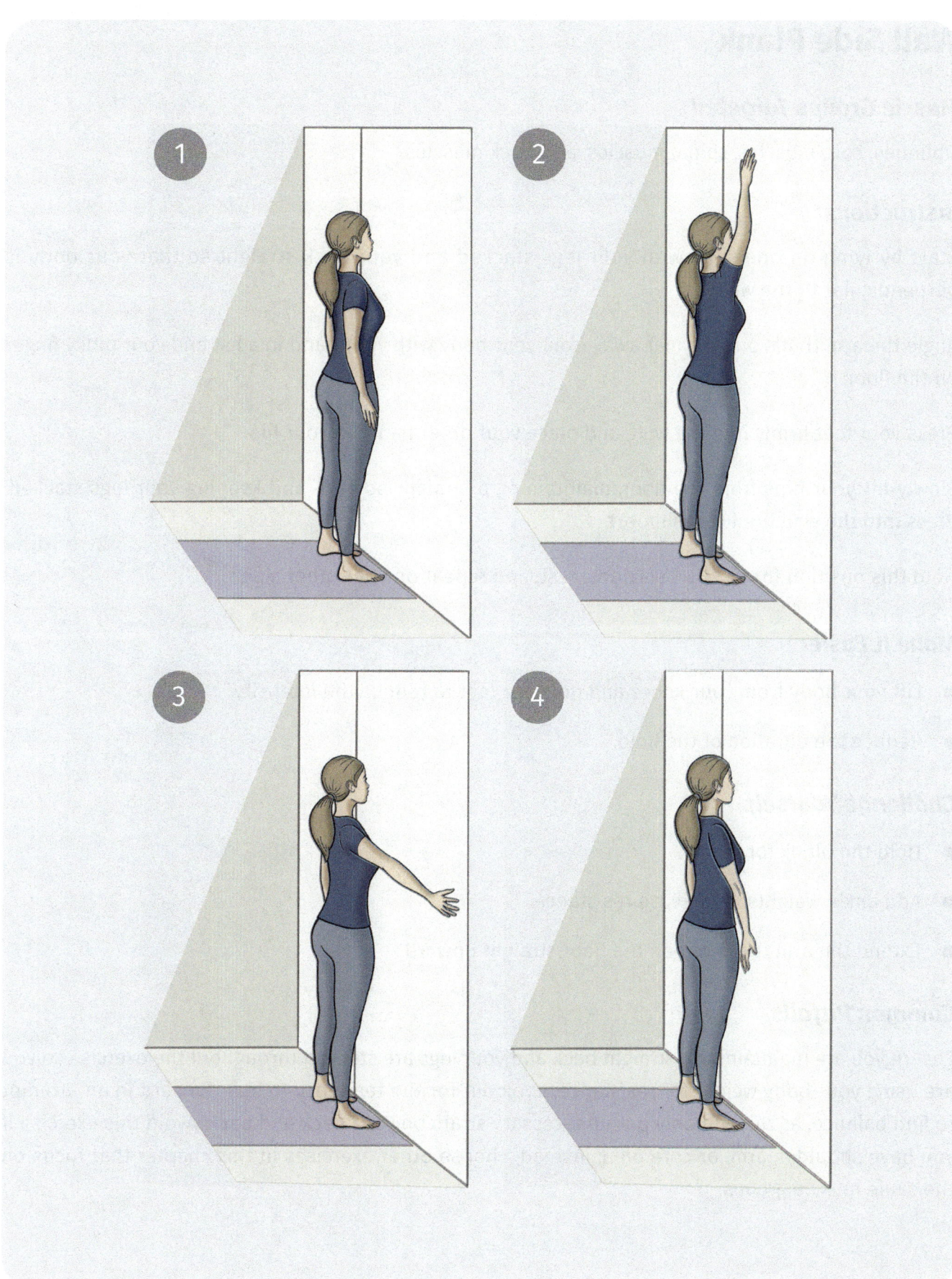

Wall Side Plank

Muscle Groups Targeted

Obliques, core muscles, spinal muscles, and back muscles.

Instructions

Start by lying on one side, with your legs stacked and your back straight so that your body is perpendicular to the wall.

Angle the arm that's on your mat away from your body with your hand in a fist and your pinky finger on the floor.

Press your feet firmly into the wall, and place your other hand on your hip.

Slowly lift your hips from the floor, maintaining a straight posture and keeping your legs stacked. Press into the wall firmly for support.

Hold this position for up to 30 seconds, rest, and repeat on your other side.

Make It Easier

- Lift your body from your knees and not your feet to reduce the intensity.
- Reduce the duration of the hold.

Challenge Yourself

- Hold the plank for longer.
- Add ankle weights to increase resistance.
- Extend the arm that's not on the floor straight upward.

Common Pitfalls

Ensure you are maintaining a straight back and your legs are stacked throughout the exercise so you are using your body weight for resistance. Look out for the tendency to lean forward in an attempt to find balance, as this will only put unnecessary strain on your neck and back. Avoid this exercise if you have shoulder, arm, or core pain; instead, choose other exercises in this chapter that focus on the same muscle groups.

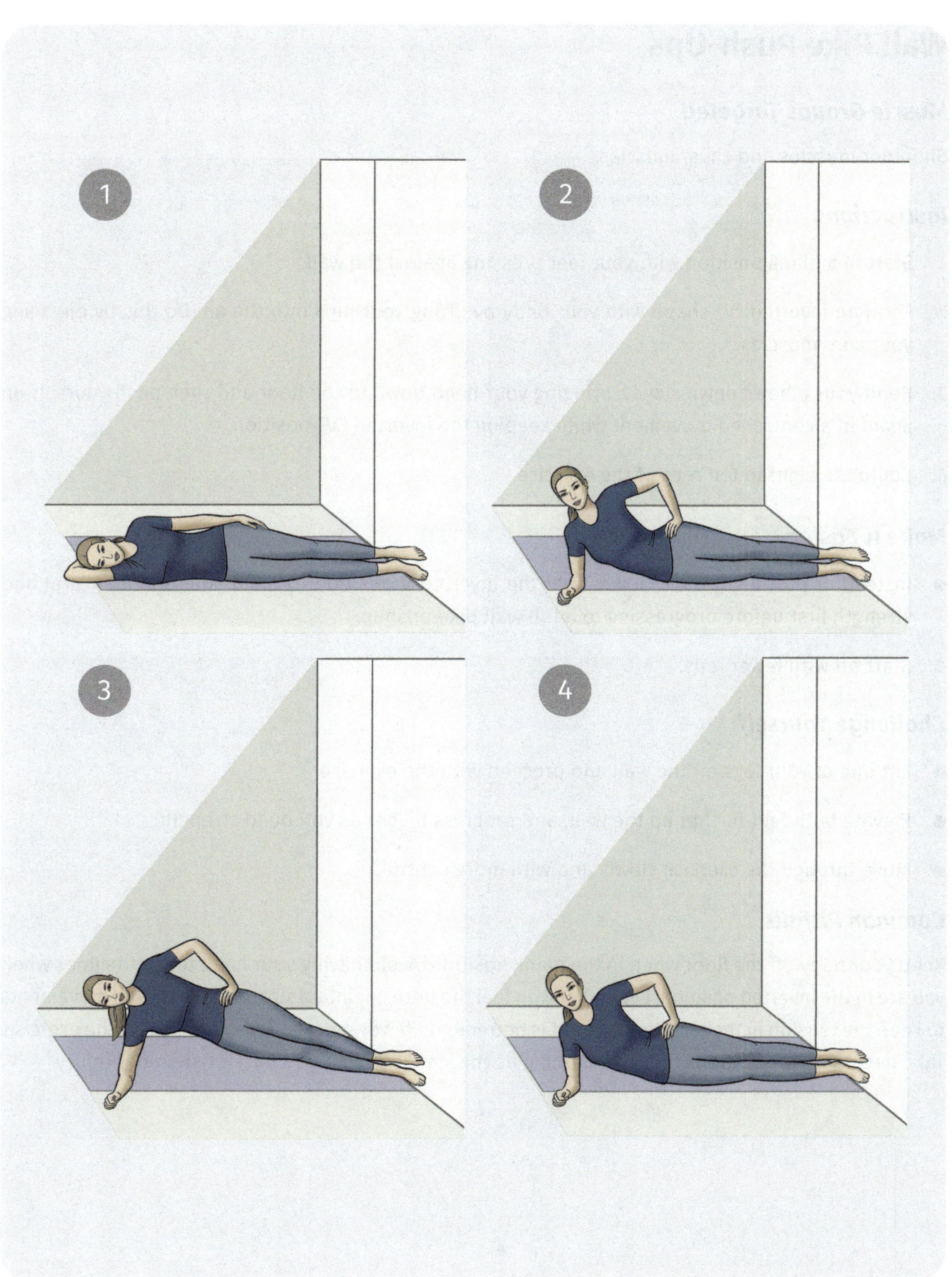

Wall Pike Push-Ups

Muscle Groups Targeted

Shoulder muscles and chest muscles.

Instructions

1. Start in a plank position with your feet pressing against the wall.

2. Form an inverted "V" shape with your body by lifting your hips into the air. Do this by engaging your core muscles.

3. Bend your elbows down slowly, bringing your head down to the floor and then push yourself up again in a controlled movement while keeping the inverted "V" position.

4. Complete eight to ten reps of the exercise.

Make It Easier

- Instead of pushing up and down, hold the inverted V position to build your shoulder arm and strength first before progressing to a full wall pike pushup.

- Start off with fewer reps.

Challenge Yourself

- Lift one of your legs off the wall and proceed with the exercise.

- Elevate both feet further up the wall, and progress higher as you build strength.

- Move through the exercise slowly and with more control.

Common Pitfalls

Keep your body off the floor when in the plank position. Avoid having your head touch the floor when you are in the inverted position. Even when you feel the burn, maintain slow and controlled movements to keep the tension in the target muscles. It is better to do fewer reps than to rush through the exercise. Take necessary precautions to avoid slipping as this can lead to a bad back or shoulder injury.

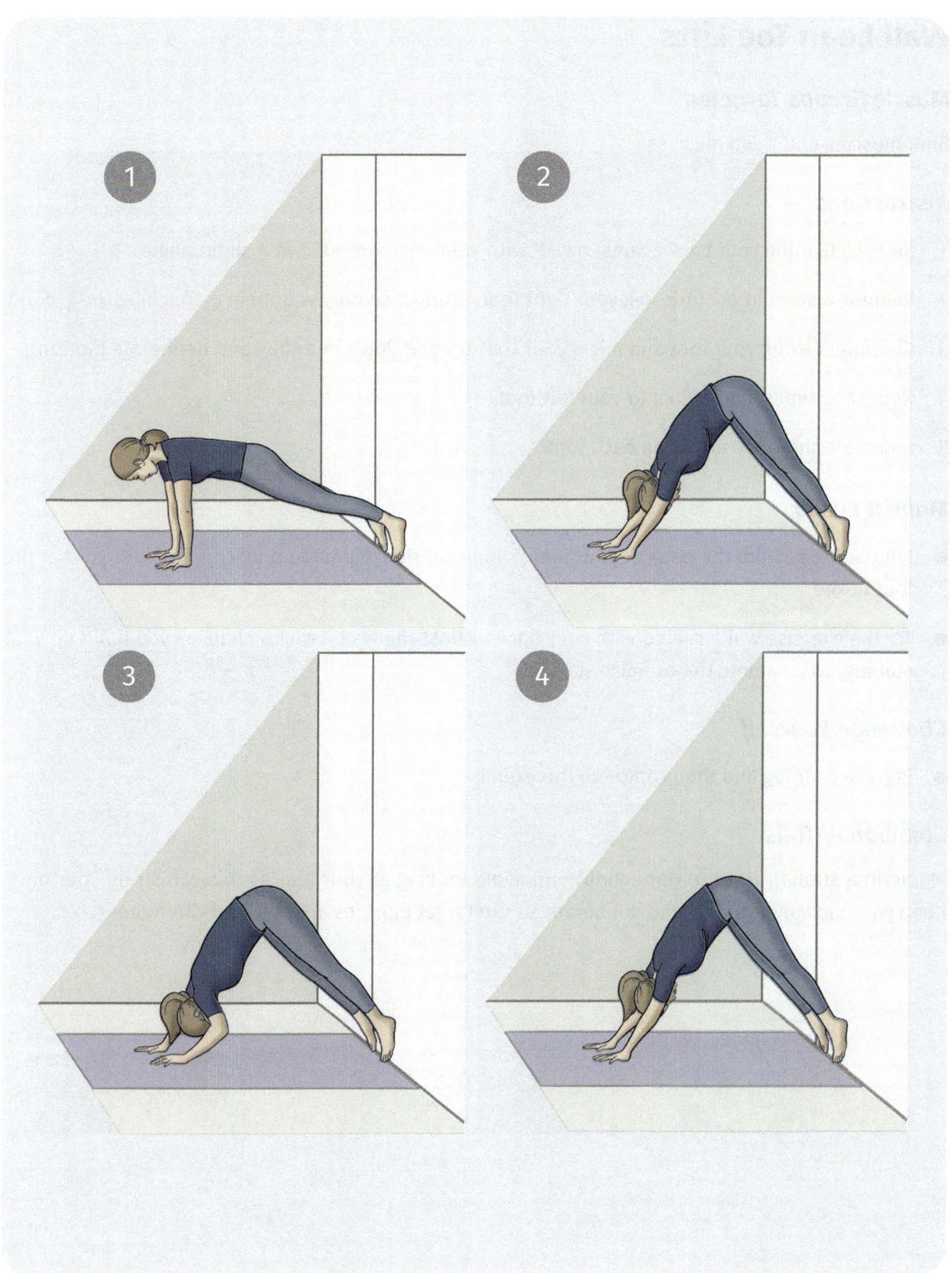

Wall Lean Toe Lifts

Muscle Groups Targeted

Shin muscles and thigh muscles.

Instructions

1. Start by leaning your back against a wall with your legs extended at a slight angle.

2. Keeping a straight posture, flex your right foot, lifting it so only your heel is touching the ground.

3. Continue flexing your foot and move your toes up and down in a slow and deliberate motion.

4. Repeat 10 times, and switch to your left foot.

5. Complete three reps of 10 on each foot.

Make It Easier

- Lift your toes from the balls of your feet if you experience pain and discomfort with your entire foot flexed.

- Try the exercise while seated with your back against the wall, or on a chair, as you build up your stability to complete the exercise standing.

Challenge Yourself

- Elevate your leg and then complete the exercise.

Common Pitfalls

Maintain a straight posture throughout and avoid looking at your feet as this can strain your neck. Keep your movements slow and deliberate so the target muscles are engaged throughout.

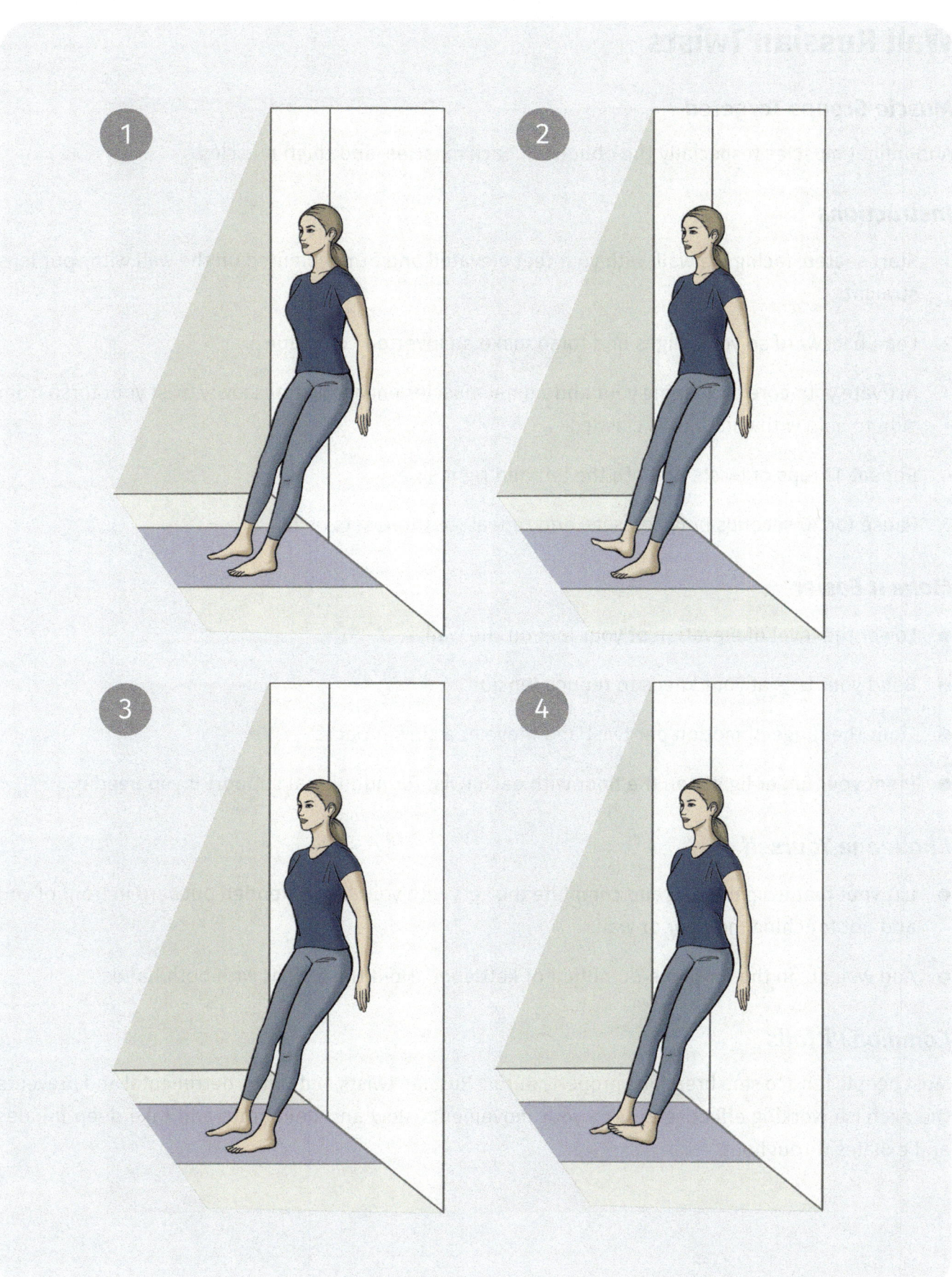

Wall Russian Twists

Muscle Groups Targeted

Abdominal muscles (especially the obliques), back muscles, and thigh muscles.

Instructions

1. Start seated, facing the wall, with your feet elevated and firmly planted on the wall with your legs straight.

2. Lean backward so your thighs and torso make an inverted "V" shape.

3. Activate your core by keeping your abdominal muscles engaged, then slowly twist your torso from side to side with your hands clasped.

4. Repeat 12 reps of twists on both the left and right side.

5. Pause for 30 seconds between sets, and repeat for three sets of 12.

Make It Easier

- Lower the level of elevation of your feet on the wall.
- Bend your legs at your knees to reduce tension.
- Limit the range of motion per twist and move at a slower pace.
- Plant your finger lightly on the floor with each twist for additional support if you need it.

Challenge Yourself

- Lift your feet from the wall and complete the sets with your legs extended outward in front of you and not touching the floor or wall.
- Add weights in the form of a dumbbell or kettlebell. Hold the weight with both hands.

Common Pitfalls

Most people tend to stop breathing properly during Russian twists, but this is detrimental and prevents the exercise working effectively. Keep your movements slow and deliberate and take deep inhales and exhales throughout.

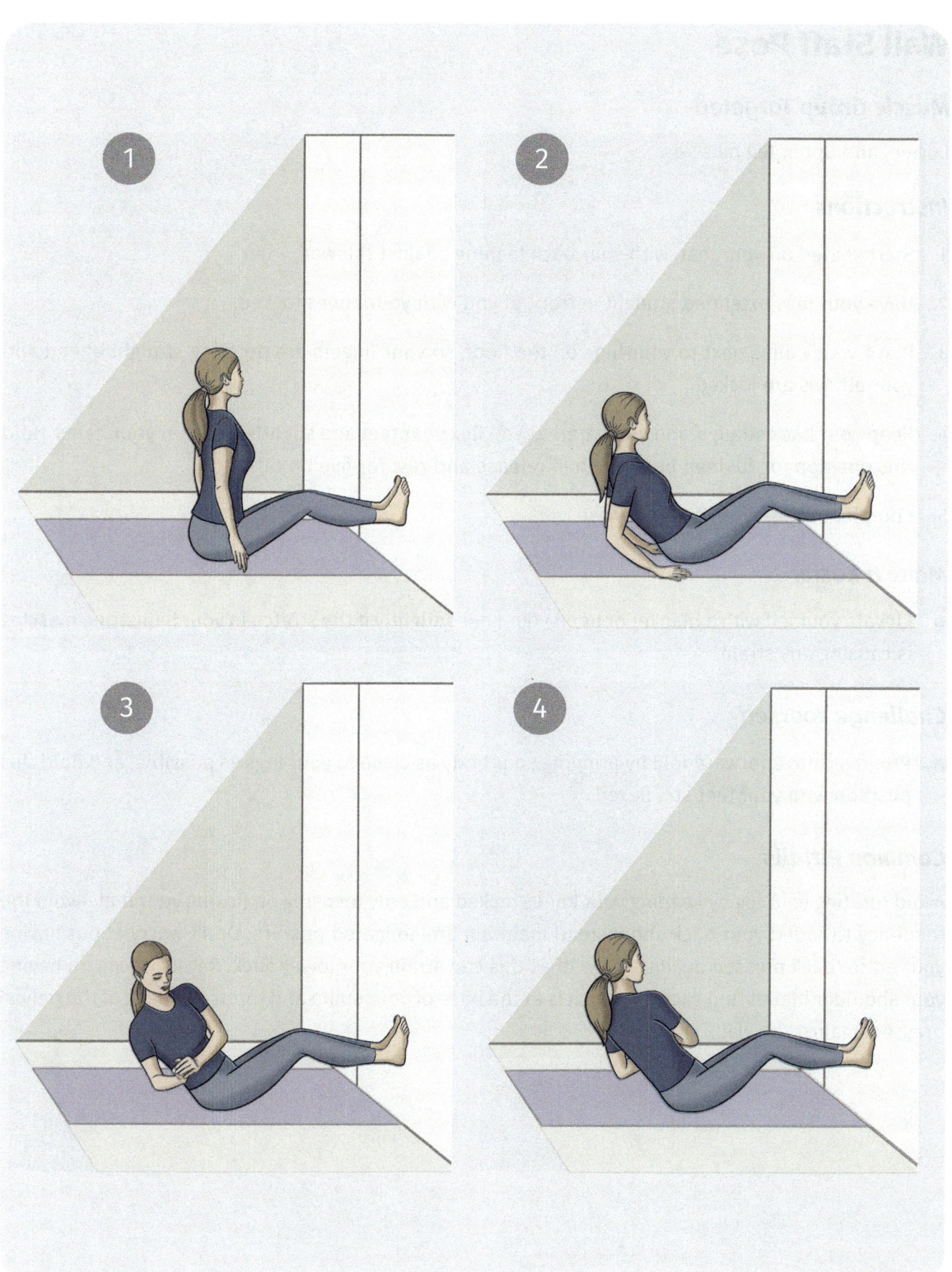

Wall Staff Pose

Muscle Group Targeted

Lower- and upper leg muscles.

Instructions

1. Start seated on your mat, with your back leaning against the wall.

2. Have your legs extended straight in front of you with your knees locked.

3. Place your palms next to your hips on the floor, so your fingers are pointing straight ahead and your elbows are locked.

4. Keep your back straight and elongated as you flex your feet and slightly rotate at your heels. Hold this position for 10 deep breaths, then release and rest for five breaths.

5. Complete three reps of the exercise.

Make It Easier

- Elevate yourself with a blanket or bend your knees slightly if the stretch in your hamstring muscles is causing any strain.

Challenge Yourself

- Progress into a forward fold by bringing your body as close to your legs as possible, and hold this position with your feet still flexed.

Common Pitfalls

Avoid rotating your leg by keeping your knees locked and only focusing on flexing your feet. Avoid the tendency to round your back and instead maintain an elongated posture. Don't worry about having your entire back pressed against the wall as this can strain your lower back. Rather, focus on having your shoulder blades and sacrum (which is at the base of your spine and forms the back of the pelvis) pressed against the wall.

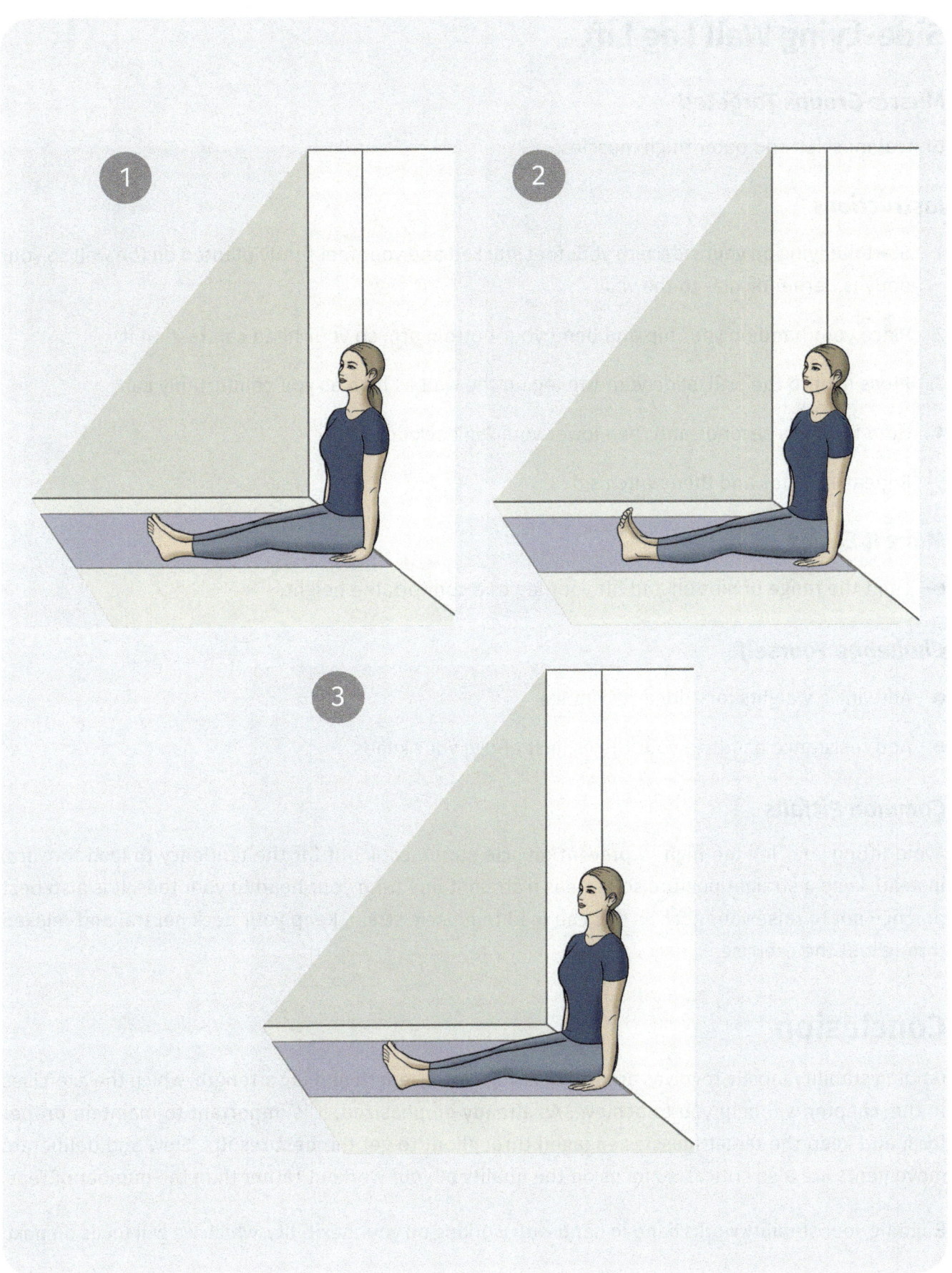

WALL PILATES WORKOUTS FOR WOMEN | 69

Side-Lying Wall Leg Lift

Muscle Groups Targeted

Gluteal muscles and outer thigh muscles.

Instructions

1. Start out lying on your side with your feet stacked and your feet firmly planted on the wall so your body is perpendicular to the wall.

2. Place your hand on your hip and bend your bottom arm so your head can rest on it.

3. Pressing into the wall, slide your top leg up the wall as high as you comfortably can.

4. Hold for a few seconds and then lower your leg back down.

5. Repeat 10 times and then switch sides.

Make It Easier

- Limit the range of motion and lift your leg to a comfortable height.

Challenge Yourself

- Add ankle weights for added resistance.
- Add resistance bands to your thighs, just above your knees.

Common Pitfalls

Avoid lifting your leg too high to prevent muscle strain. Look out for the tendency to lean forward; instead, keep a straight posture so there is a straight line from your head to your toes. It is also best practice not to raise your neck as this can lead to muscle strain. Keep your neck neutral and relaxed throughout the exercise.

Conclusion

Gaining stability mostly revolves around building core strength and leg strength, which the exercises in this chapter will help you to achieve. As already emphasized, it is important to maintain proper form and keep the target muscles engaged throughout to get the best results. Slow and deliberate movements are also critical, so focus on the quality of your workout rather than the number of reps.

Building your stability works hand in hand with working on your flexibility, which we will focus on next.

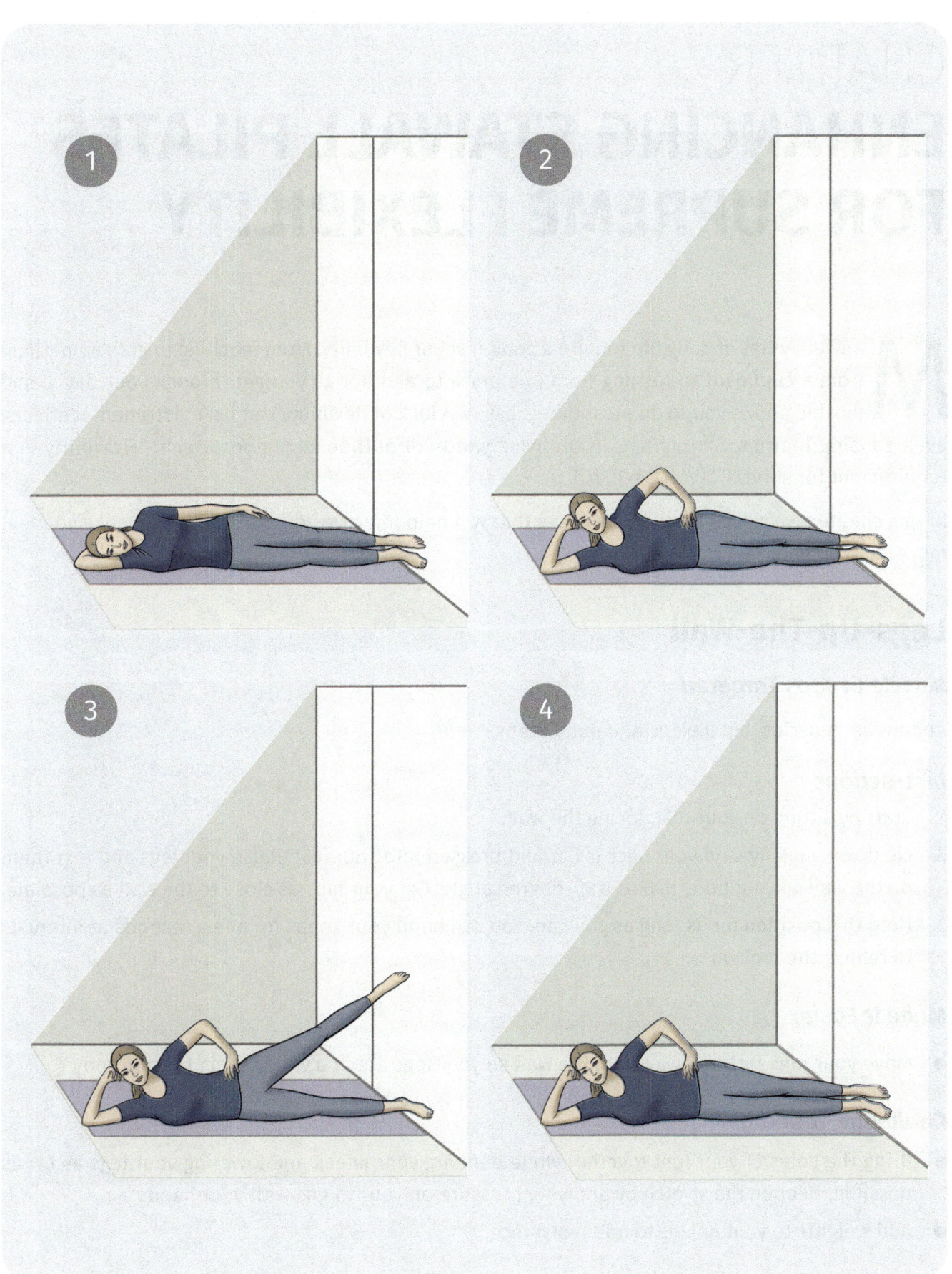

CHAPTER 7
ENHANCING STAWALL PILATES FOR SUPREME FLEXIBILITY

Many activities of daily life require a good level of flexibility. From reaching to grab something from a cupboard to rushing from one place to another as you get through your day, being flexible allows you to do most things easily. A lack of flexibility can have detrimental effects, even causing injuries. Simply put, in the wise words of author Rogen Von Oech, "Flexibility is a requirement for survival" (Von Oech, n.d.).

In this chapter, we will go through exercises that will help improve your flexibility and make you feel more agile on your feet.

Legs-Up-The-Wall

Muscle Groups Targeted
Abdominal muscles, hip flexors, and quadriceps.

Instructions
1. Start by sitting on your mat, facing the wall.
2. Lie down, making sure your back is flat and pressed into your mat. Raise your legs and rest them on the wall so your body makes a 90-degree angle. Get your hips as close to the wall as possible.
3. Hold this position for as long as you can. You can bend your knees for a few seconds at intervals to relieve the tension.

Make It Easier
- Move your hips further away from the wall so your legs are at a wider angle to your body.

Challenge Yourself
- Bring the soles of your feet together while bending your knees and lowering your legs as far as possible. Deepen the stretch by applying pressure on your thighs with your hands.
- Add weights to your ankles to add resistance.
- Cross your legs over each other in scissor kicks while they are up against the wall.

Common Pitfalls
Resist the urge to arch your back as this can cause discomfort in your lower back (Cronkleton, 2020).

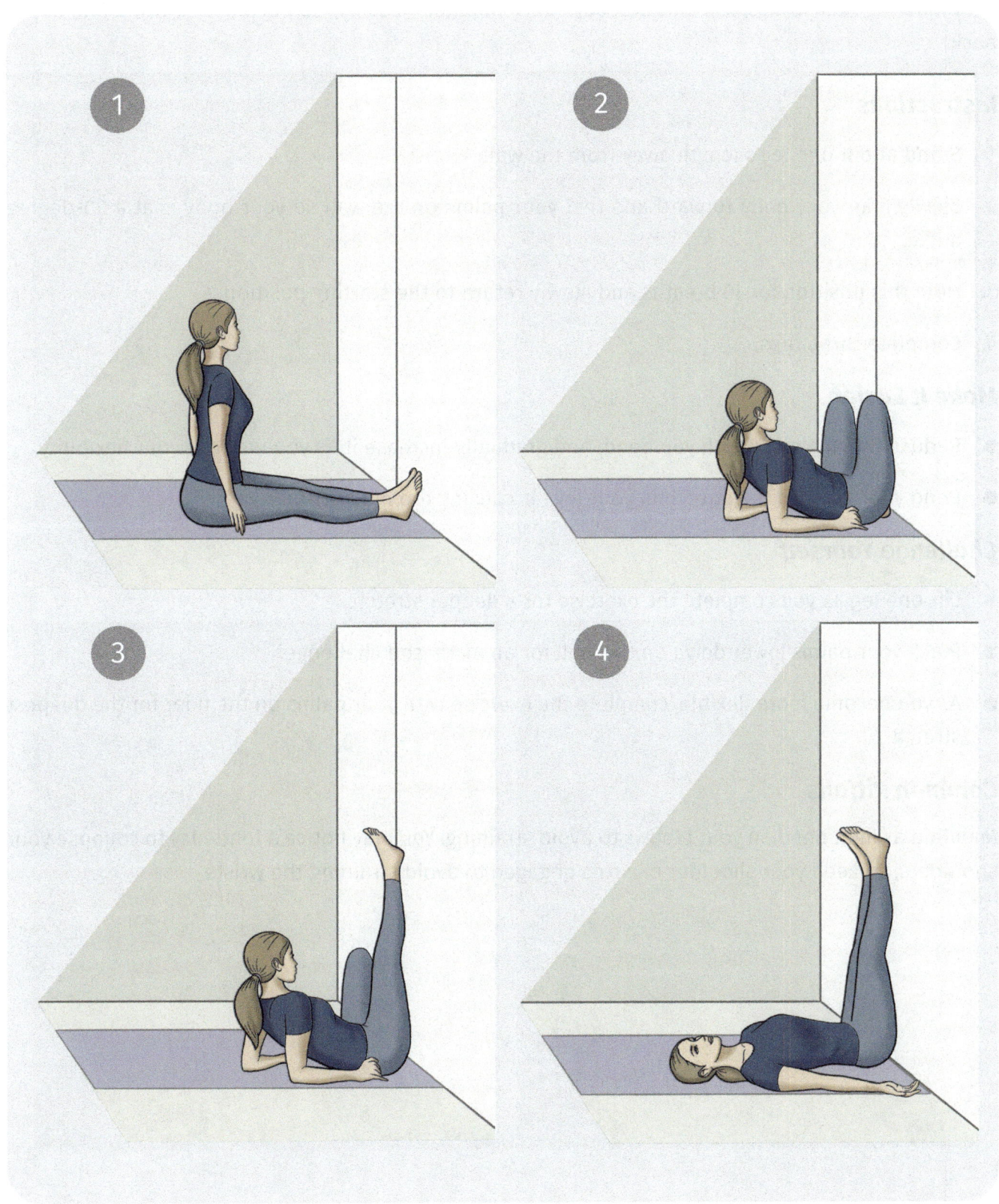

Wall Downward Facing Dog

Muscle Groups Targeted

Core muscles, hamstrings, calf muscles, deltoids (shoulder muscles), spinal muscles, arms, and upper back.

Instructions

1. Stand about one leg's length away from the wall.

2. Slowly lean your body forward and rest your palms on the wall so your body is at a 90-degree angle.

3. Hold this position for 10 breaths and slowly return to the starting position.

4. Complete three reps.

Make It Easier

- Reduce the angle at which you bend, and gradually increase it as you improve your flexibility.

- Bend your knees if the stretch in your legs is causing too much strain.

Challenge Yourself

- Lift one leg as you complete the exercise for a deeper stretch.

- Place your palms lower down on the wall for an increased challenge.

- As you become more flexible, complete the exercise with your palms on the floor for the deepest stretch.

Common Pitfalls

Maintain a slight bend on your elbows to avoid straining. You may notice a tendency to collapse your shoulders, so keep your shoulder muscles engaged to avoid straining the wrists.

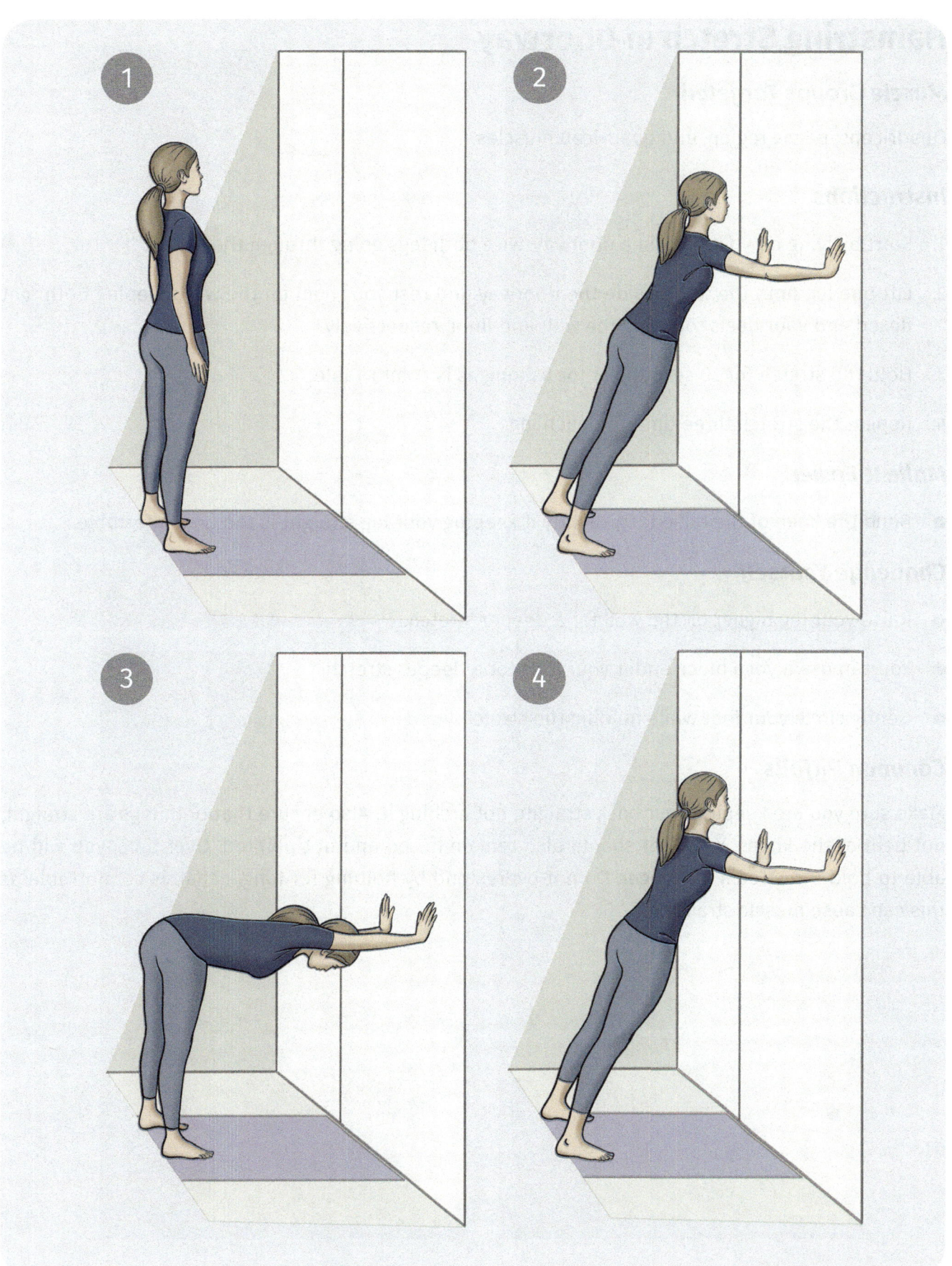

Hamstring Stretch in Doorway

Muscle Groups Targeted

Quadriceps, pelvic region, and quadricep muscles.

Instructions

1. Start by lying on your back in a doorway, with both legs going through the door.

2. Lift one leg onto the wall beside the doorway and rest your heel on the wall, keeping both feet flexed and your heels touching the wall and floor, respectively.

3. Hold the stretch for 30 seconds or for as long as is comfortable.

4. Repeat the stretch three times on each leg.

Make It Easier

- Bend the knee of the raised leg slightly if keeping your leg straight is too uncomfortable.

Challenge Yourself

- Raise your leg higher on the wall for a deeper stretch.

- You can use a yoga block under your hips for a deeper stretch.

- Gently circle your foot while holding the stretch.

Common Pitfalls

Make sure you are keeping your back straight, not arching it. Also ensure that both legs are straight, not bent at the knees. Your feet should also remain flexed and not pointed. Over time, you will be able to hold the stretch for longer. Do not overextend by holding for longer than is comfortable as this can cause muscle strain.

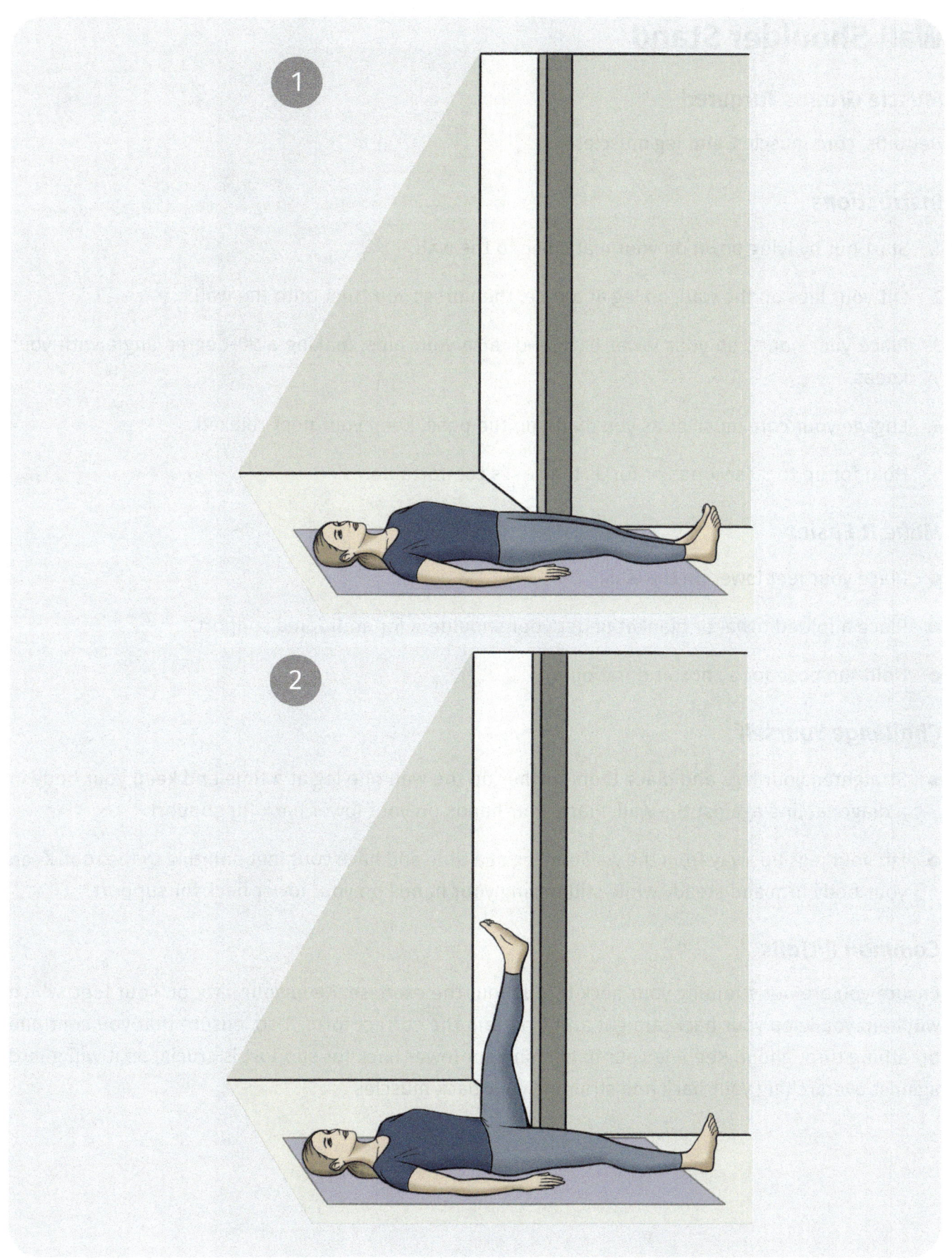

WALL PILATES WORKOUTS FOR WOMEN | 77

Wall Shoulder Stand

Muscle Groups Targeted

Deltoids, core muscles, and leg muscles.

Instructions

1. Start out by lying down on your mat close to the wall.
2. Lift your legs on the wall, on leg at a time, then press your feet onto the wall.
3. Place your hands on your lower back and raise your hips, making a 90-degree angle with your knees.
4. Engage your core muscles as you maintain the pose. Keep your neck relaxed.
5. Hold for up to 30 seconds or for as long as is comfortable.

Make It Easier

- Place your feet lower on the wall.
- Place a folded towel or blanket under your shoulders for additional support.
- Hold the pose for a shorter duration.

Challenge Yourself

- Straighten your legs and place them further up the wall one leg at a time and keep your body in a diagonal line against the wall. Place your hands on your lower back for support.
- Lift your legs up away from the wall one leg at a time and have your feet pointing to the roof. Keep your body firm and steady while still having your hands on your lower back for support.

Common Pitfalls

Ensure you are not straining your neck throughout the exercise. Keep your gaze on your feet, which will help you keep your back straight and maintain the correct form. Also, ensure that you continue breathing throughout. Keeping your hands on your lower back for support is crucial as it will guard against overarching your back and straining your back muscles.

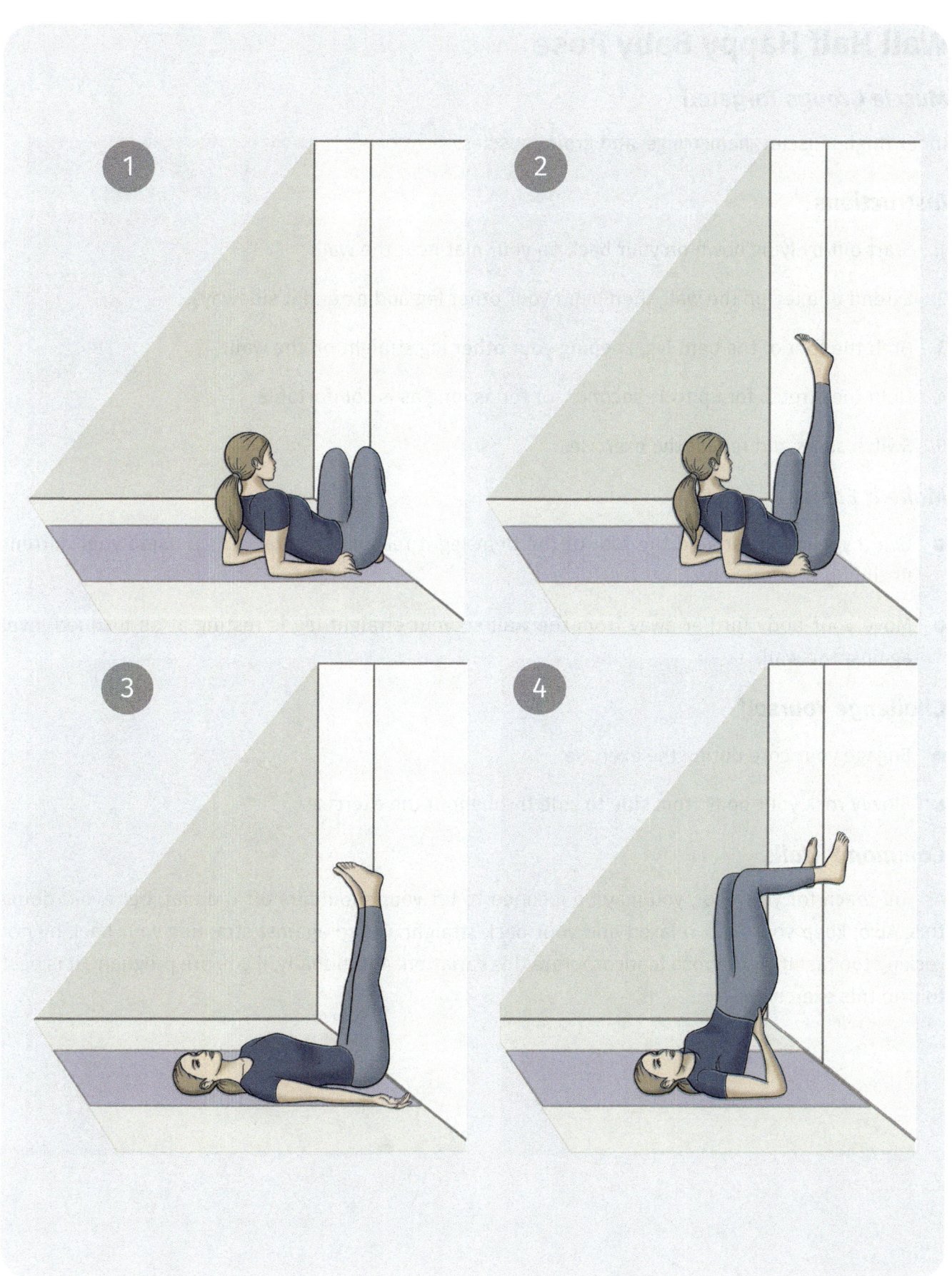

Wall Half Happy Baby Pose

Muscle Groups Targeted

Inner thigh muscles, hamstrings, and groin muscles.

Instructions

1. Start out by lying down on your back on your mat near the wall.

2. Extend one leg up the wall, then bend your other leg and extend it sideways.

3. Grab the foot of the bent leg, keeping your other leg straight on the wall.

4. Hold the stretch for up to 15 seconds, or for as long as is comfortable.

5. Switch sides and repeat the exercise.

Make It Easier

- Use a yoga strap around the foot of the bent leg if reaching to grab it is outside your current flexibility comfort zone.

- Move your body further away from the wall so your straight leg is resting at an inclined level against the wall.

Challenge Yourself

- Engage your core during the exercise.

- Slowly rock your body from side to side throughout the exercise.

Common Pitfalls

As you reach for your foot, you may be inclined to lift your shoulders off the mat, but avoid doing this. Also, keep your neck relaxed and your back straight. Guard against straining your back by not rocking too fast if you choose to incorporate this variation. Additionally, if you are pregnant, it is best to skip this exercise.

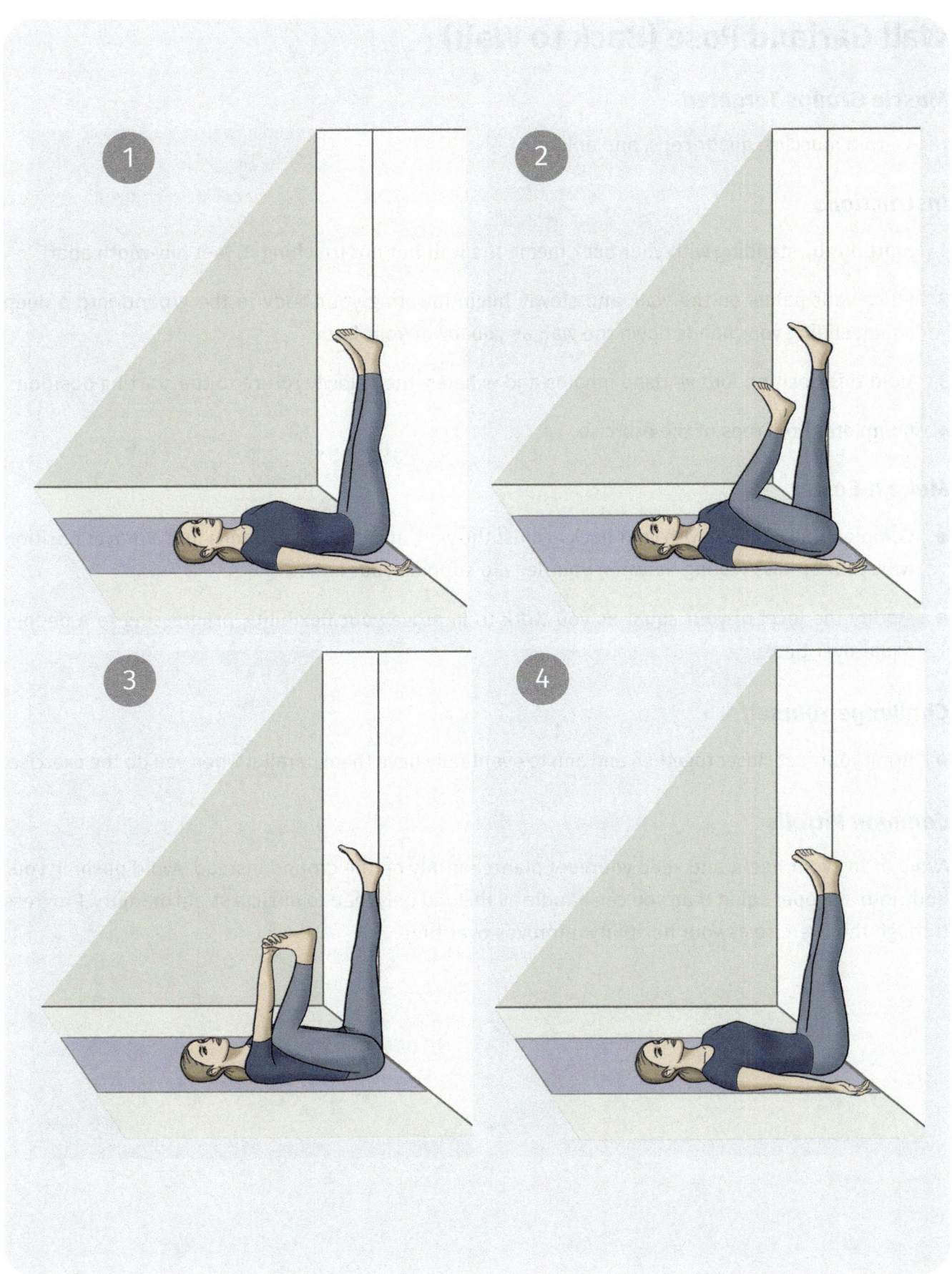

Wall Garland Pose (Back to Wall)

Muscle Groups Targeted

Hips, groin muscles, quadriceps, and ankles.

Instructions

1. Start out by standing with your back facing the wall but not touching it, feet hip-width apart.

2. Place your palms on the wall, and slowly begin lowering your body to the ground into a deep squat, sliding your hands down the wall as you lower your body.

3. Hold this position for five deep inhales and exhales, then slowly return to the starting position.

4. Complete three reps of the exercise.

Make It Easier

- Complete the exercise with your back against the wall, and bring your hands into a prayer position with your elbows resting between your legs to support your knees.

- Modify the level of your squat as you work to improve your flexibility, progressing to a deeper squat over time.

Challenge Yourself

- Bring your feet closer together, and aim to eventually have them parallel when you do the exercise.

Common Pitfalls

Avoid lifting your heels, and keep your feet planted firmly on the ground instead. Avoid pushing your body into a deeper squat than you can handle as this will only lead to muscle strain or injury. Progress through the exercise as your flexibility improves over time.

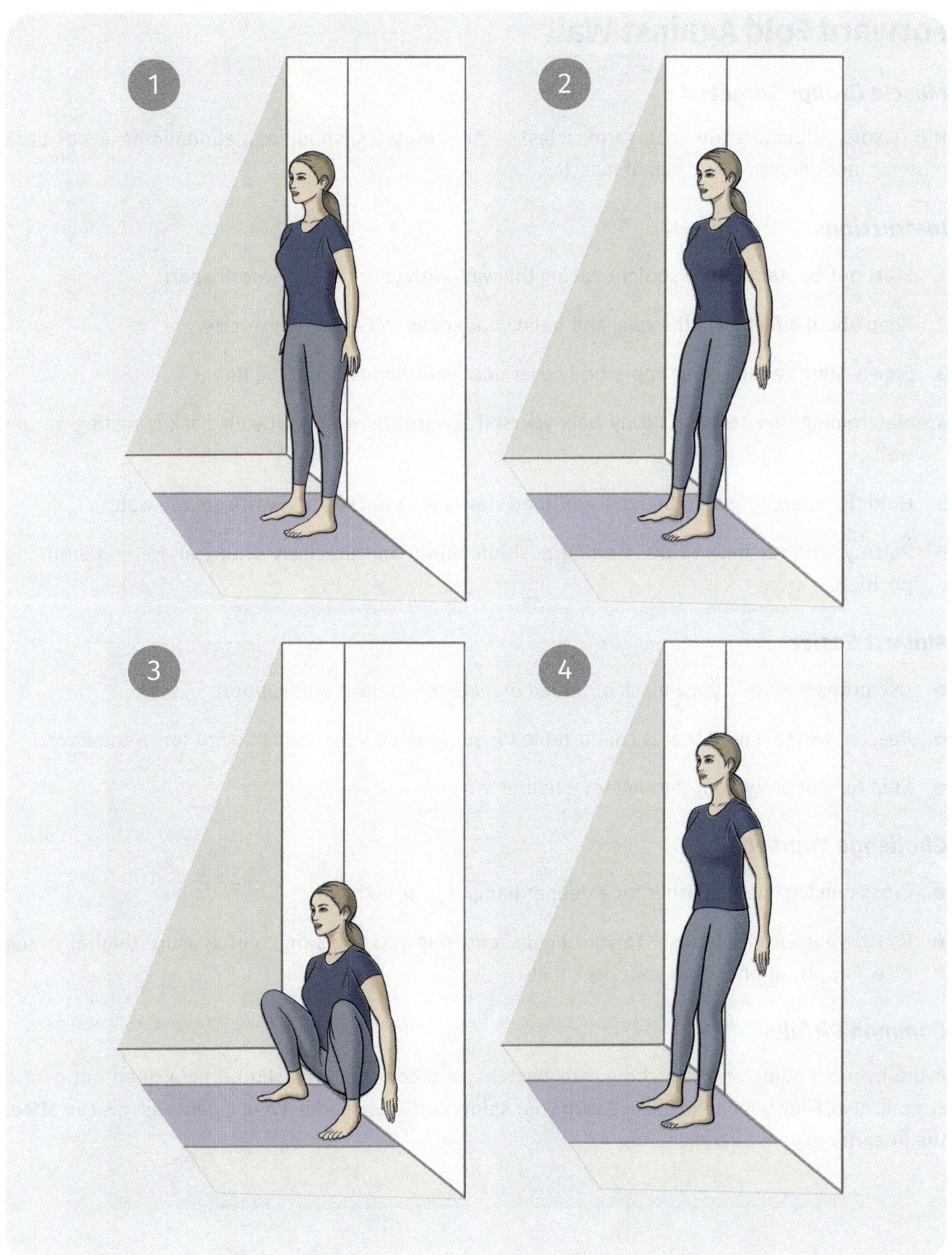

WALL PILATES WORKOUTS FOR WOMEN | 83

Forward Fold Against Wall

Muscle Groups Targeted

Hip flexors, adductors (inner thigh muscles), gluteal muscles, shoulders, abdominals, lower back muscles, neck muscles, and spinal muscles.

Instructions

1. Start out by standing up straight, facing the wall, with your feet hip-width apart.
2. Keep about 3 feet from the wall, and bend your knees to begin the exercise.
3. Slowly start bending your upper body over until your hands reach the floor.
4. Maintaining this posture, slowly walk yourself toward the wall until your back is resting on the wall.
5. Hold the stretch for 5–10 breaths, and then slowly walk backward away from the wall.
6. Raise your body back to the starting position slowly and precisely until you are in a standing position.

Make It Easier

- Use props such as a yoga block or folded blanket for comfort and support.
- Reach down to a level that is comfortable for you, even if your hands do not touch the floor.
- Step further away from the wall for a lighter stretch.

Challenge Yourself

- Cross one leg over the other for a deeper hamstring stretch.
- Reach your forehead closer to your knees, ensuring you focus on comfort more than anything else. Pay attention to how your neck feels.

Common Pitfalls

Avoid overextending and stretching your back beyond comfort. This should be a deep but gentle stretch. Also, keep your head aligned with your spine, and avoid sudden movements as this can affect the integrity of your straight spine.

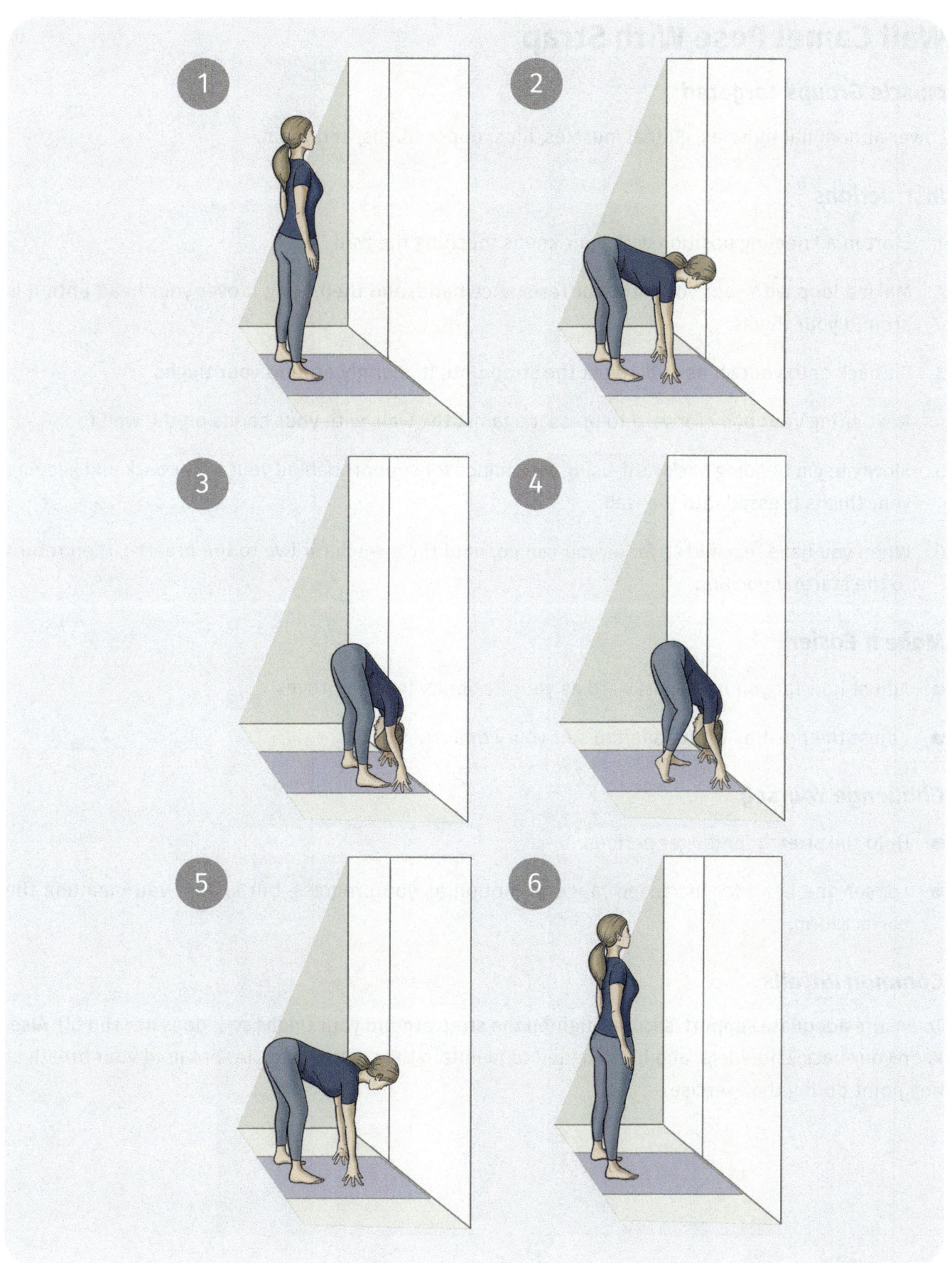

Wall Camel Pose With Strap

Muscle Groups Targeted

Lower abdominal muscles, gluteal muscles, hips, upper thighs, and groin.

Instructions

1. Start in a kneeling position with your knees touching the wall.

2. Make a loop with your yoga strap or resistance band, and then bring it over your head until it is around your thighs.

3. Sit back onto your shins and adjust the strap until it is firmly around your thighs.

4. Next, bring your body forward to press it against the wall, with your hands on the wall too.

5. Slowly begin bending backward, using your hands for support behind your lower back and keeping your thighs pressed into the wall.

6. When you have reached as far as you can go, hold the stretch for five to ten breaths, then return to the starting position.

Make It Easier

- Adjust how far you bend backward as your flexibility level improves.
- Adjust the position of the band to suit your comfort.

Challenge Yourself

- Hold the stretch for longer periods.
- Loosen the band for increased range of motion as you progress, but ensure you maintain the correct form.

Common Pitfalls

To ensure adequate support, securely tighten the strap around your thighs so it does not slip off. Also, keep your back, shoulders, and hips aligned to maintain the correct form. Do not hold your breath at any point during the exercise.

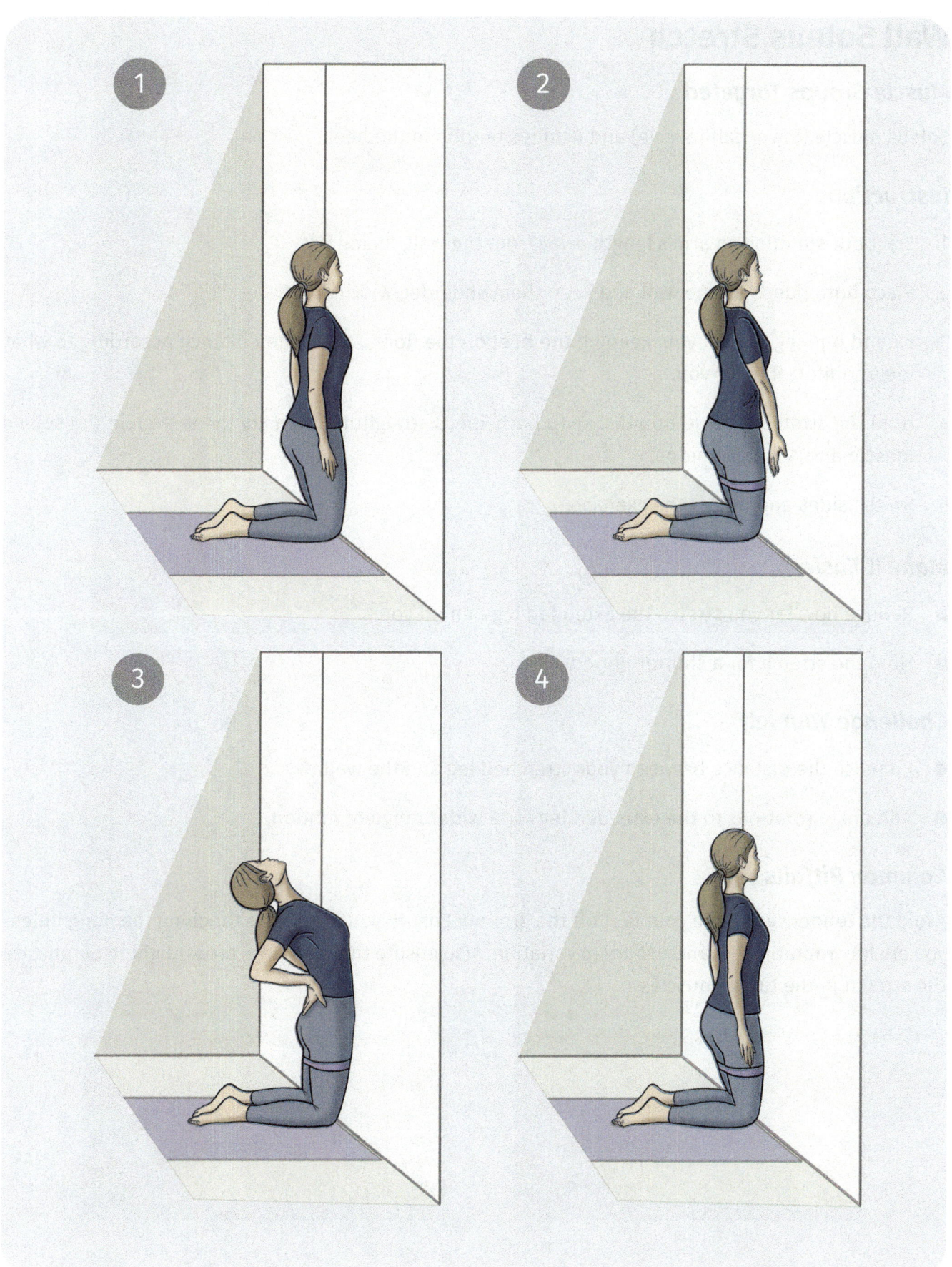

Wall Soleus Stretch

Muscle Groups Targeted

Soleus muscle (lower calf muscle) and Achilles tendon in the heel.

Instructions

1. Start out standing an arm's length away from the wall, facing it.

2. Place both hands on the wall and keep them shoulder-width apart.

3. Extend one leg behind you, keeping the heel on the floor. Adjust the distance according to what feels comfortable for you.

4. Hold the stretch for 5–10 breaths. Keep both knees straight to intensify the stretch in the soleus muscle and Achilles tendon.

5. Switch sides and repeat the exercise.

Make It Easier

- Reduce how far you stretch the extended leg behind you.
- Hold the stretch for a shorter period.

Challenge Yourself

- Increase the distance between your stretched leg and the wall.
- Add ankle rotations to the extended leg for a wider range of motion.

Common Pitfalls

Avoid the tendency to raise your feet off the ground. Ensure your heels are touching the floor, unless you are incorporating the ankle rotation variation. Also ensure that both legs are straight to emphasize the stretch in the target muscles.

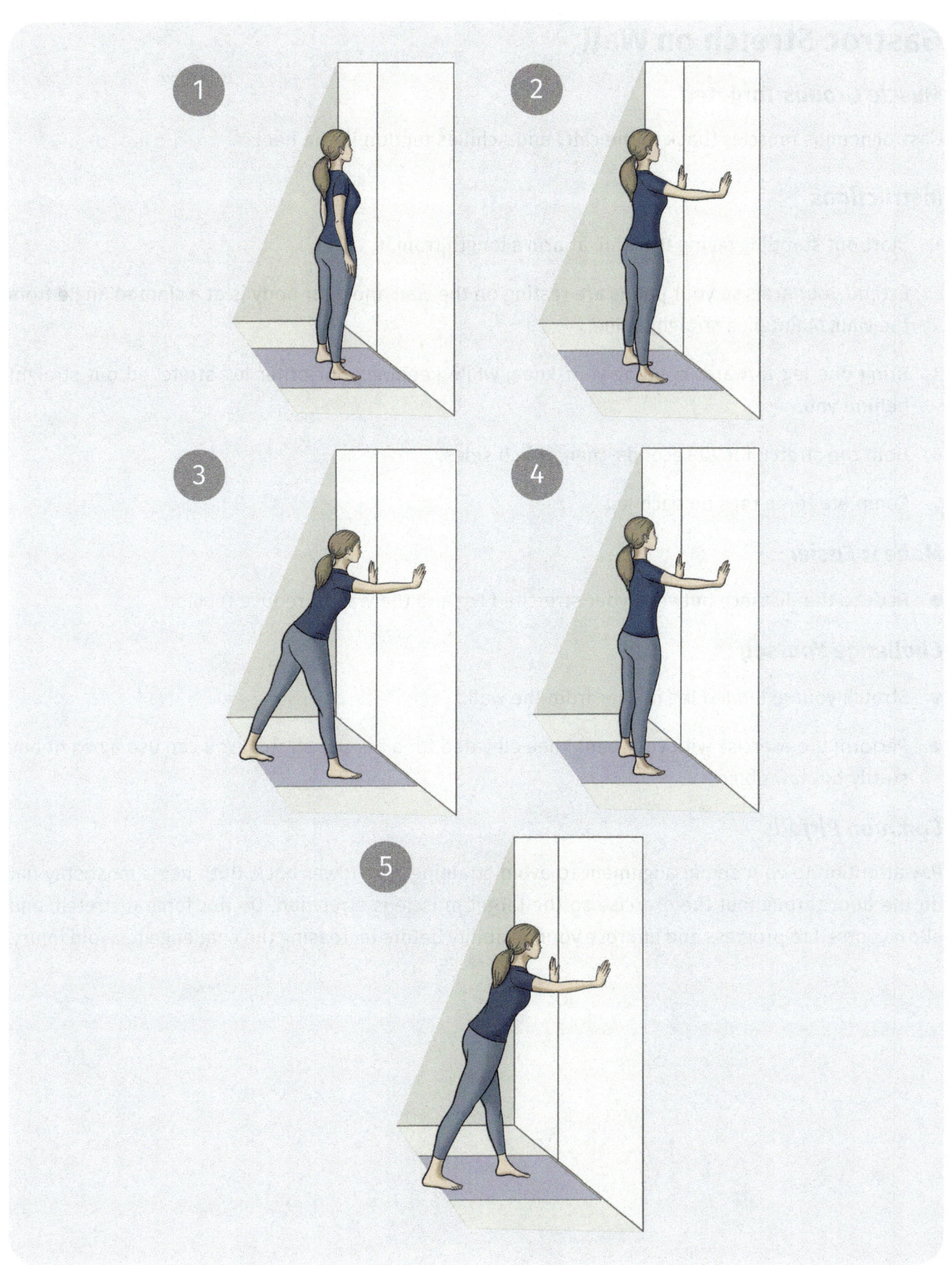

Gastroc Stretch on Wall

Muscle Groups Targeted

Gastrocnemius muscles (back of the calf) and Achilles tendon in the heel.

Instructions

1. Start out standing facing the wall, at arm's length from it.
2. Extend your arms so your palms are resting on the wall and your body is at a slanted angle from the wall. Maintain a straight spine.
3. Bring one leg forward, bending your knee, while keeping your other leg stretched out straight behind you.
4. Hold the stretch for 20 seconds, then switch sides.
5. Complete three reps on each leg.

Make It Easier

- Reduce the distance between your stretched leg and the wall to reduce tension.

Challenge Yourself

- Stretch your extended leg further from the wall.
- Perform the exercise with your bent knee elevated for a deeper stretch. You can use a box or any sturdy but low object.

Common Pitfalls

Pay attention to your spinal alignment to avoid straining your lower back. Both heels must stay flat on the floor throughout the exercise so the target muscle is stretched. Do not force a stretch, and allow yourself to progress and improve your flexibility before increasing the challenge to avoid injury.

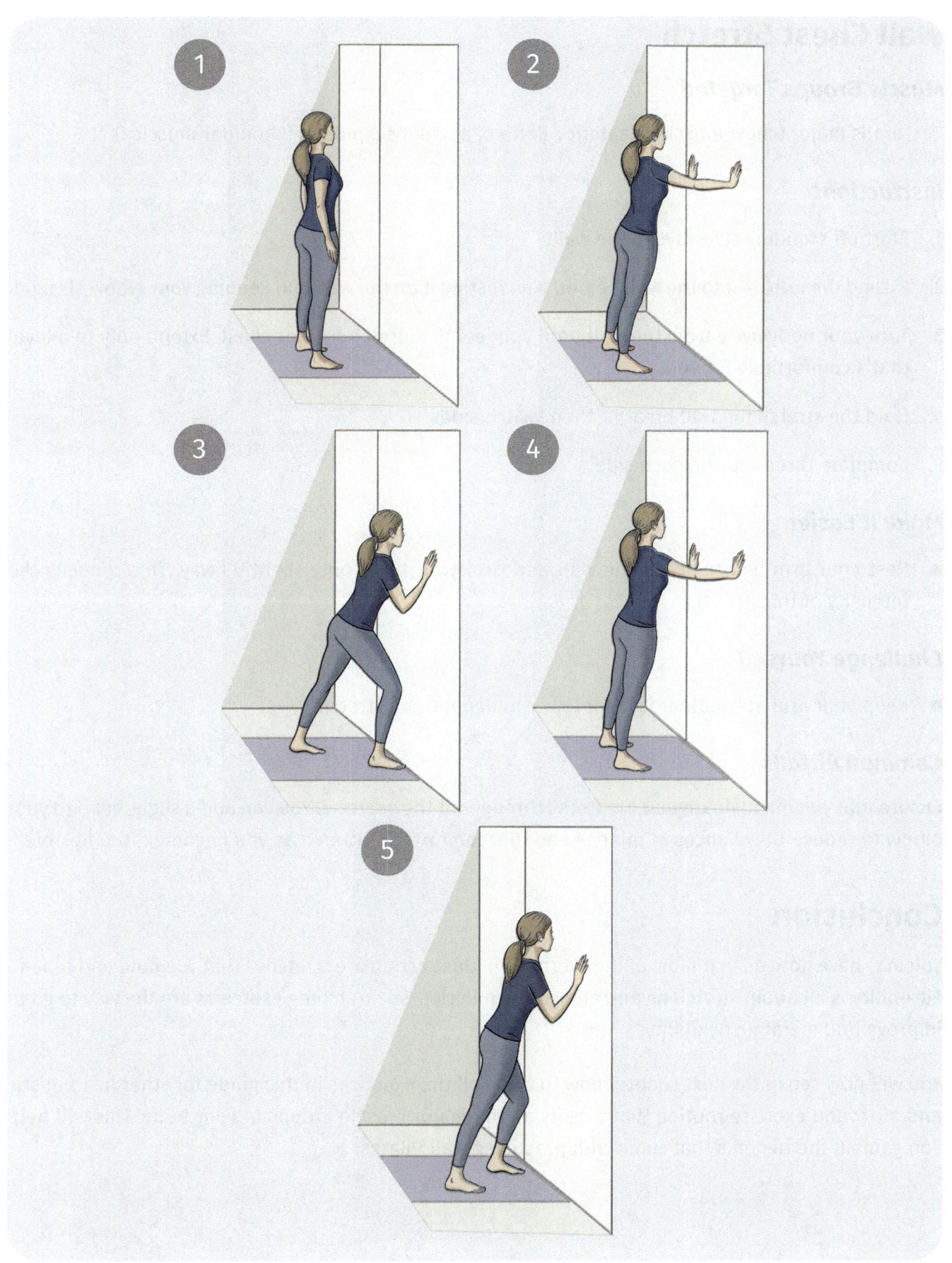

Wall Chest Stretch

Muscle Groups Targeted

Pectoralis major (chest muscles), anterior deltoid, and subscapularis (shoulder muscles).

Instructions

1. Start off standing sideways to the wall.
2. Extend the arm next to the wall behind you, resting it on the wall and keeping your elbow straight.
3. Turn your body away from the wall until you feel the stretch in your chest. Extend only to a level that's comfortable for you.
4. Hold the stretch for 5–10 breaths, then switch sides.
5. Complete three reps on each side.

Make It Easier

- Rest your arm higher up on the wall and turn your body only slightly away. This reduces the intensity of the stretch.

Challenge Yourself

- Keep your arm at shoulder level or lower to deepen the stretch.

Common Pitfalls

Ensure that you maintain regular breathing throughout the exercise. You can add a slight bend to your elbow to reduce the chances of injury. Keep to a comfortable stretch as you become more flexible.

Conclusion

You may have noticed that most of the exercises in this section are stretches that you hold and repeat. Flexibility is all about stretching and elongating muscles, so stretching exercises are the way to go to improve and maintain flexibility.

You will now see in the next chapter how to bring all the exercises in this guide together in a holistic and all-round exercise routine that targets all the major muscle groups in your body. This will help you gain all the benefits that come with practicing wall Pilates.

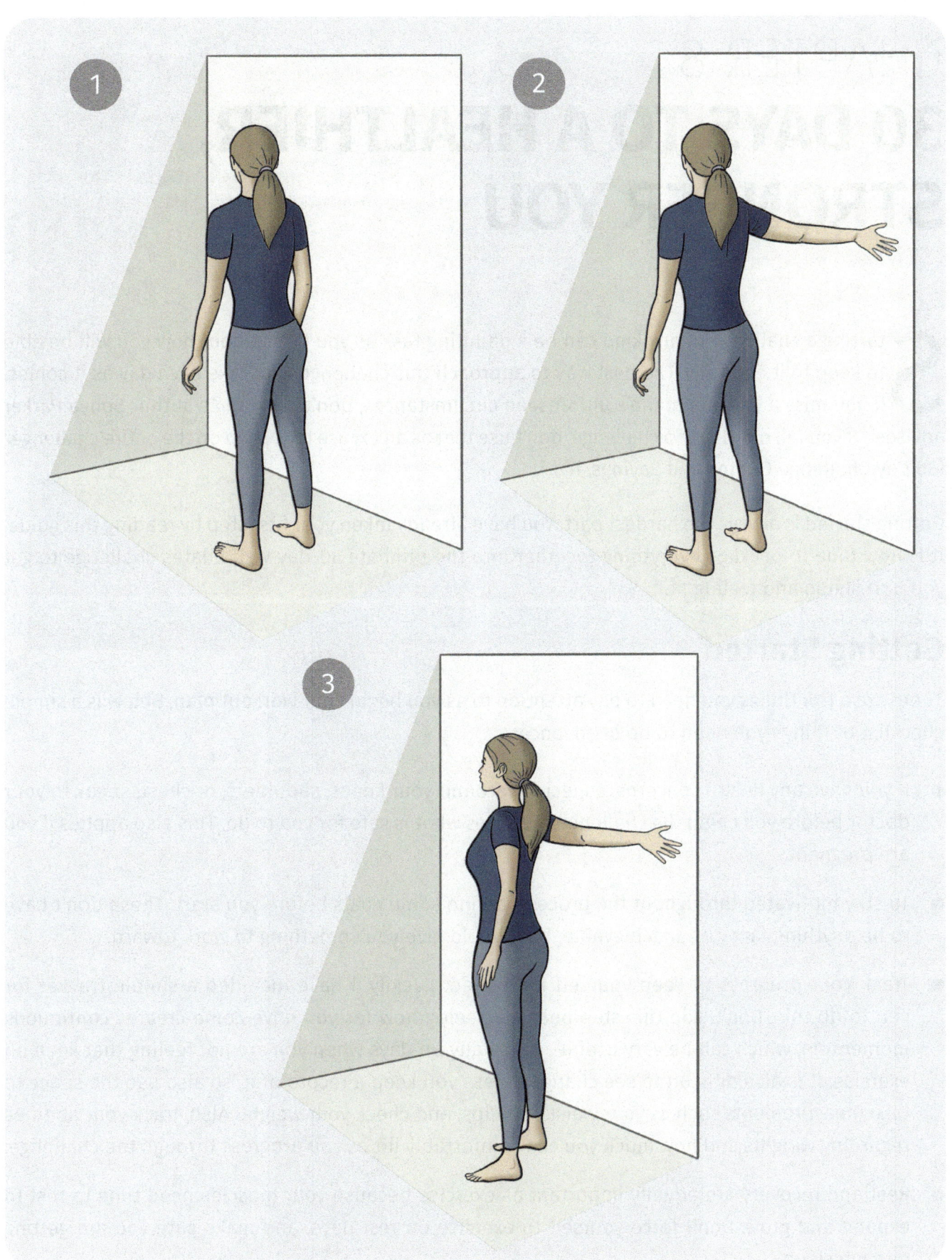

CHAPTER 8
30 DAYS TO A HEALTHIER, STRONGER YOU

Starting a challenge of any kind can be a daunting task as you think about how you will be able to keep to it each day. The best way to approach this challenge is to take each day as it comes. If you miss a day due to life's unforeseen circumstances, don't give up! As author Sonya Parker advises: "If you fail one day of a challenge, don't use that as an excuse to give up on the entire challenge" (30 Day Challenge Quotes and Sayings, n.d.).

Getting started is always the hardest part. You have already taken your first step by reading this guide. It is now time to package everything together into the ultimate 30-day wall Pilates challenge to get you into shape and feeling fit.

Getting Started

There are a few things you need to pay attention to as you begin your workout plan. Below is a simple checklist of things you need to do in advance:

- If you have any health concerns, especially around your knees, shoulders, or chest, speak to your doctor before you begin the challenge to assess what is safe for you to do. This also applies if you are pregnant.

- To stay motivated throughout the process, define some goals before you start. These don't have to be anything fancy or unachievable, but should give you something to work toward.

- Track your progress to keep yourself motivated. Luckily, I have included a simple tracker for you to do this. Don't skip this step because seeing how far you have come creates continuous momentum, which can be very useful—especially on days when you are not feeling that keen on exercise. It is also difficult to see change unless you keep a record of it, so also use the space to take measurements such as your waist and hips, and check your weight. Also, track your abilities regarding weights and how much you can comfortably lift as you progress through the challenge.

- Rest and recovery are equally important as exercise because your muscles need time to rest to expand and grow. Don't force yourself to exercise on rest days, and make sure you are getting enough sleep.

- Also crucial in muscle building and your overall health and wellness is your diet. Make sure you are feeding your body with adequate nutrients for the amount of activity you will be doing. Maintain a balanced diet, and increase your protein intake while doing strength training exercises. For cardio, you must increase your carbohydrate intake for extra energy supply. Do everything in moderation so you don't cancel out your efforts with extra calories (Mogeni, 2022).

The Workout Plan

The general structure of this program is as follows:

1. Every workout starts with a warm-up session (there is an example outlined below that you can refer to every day before starting). Warming up is important to prevent muscle strain and tears, and will ready your muscles for exertion.

2. Cardiovascular exercises come next, which will increase your heart rate and prime your body for the rest of the workout. This is also when you will burn more calories.

3. Strength training will be the next part of the exercise routine, where you can isolate different muscle groups and target different parts of the body.

4. The final stage of the workout routine will incorporate exercises for flexibility and stability.

5. Finally, you will stretch and cool down, which is an important part of the routine that should also never be skipped. This helps your muscles recover and reduces the chances of feeling pain a few hours after completing a routine.

Each workout will take 30–45 minutes, so ensure you allocate enough time per day to complete the exercises. The best part is that you will not notice the time go by as you will be busy getting through the program, so don't feel overwhelmed by this estimated duration. The duration of your workout will also differ depending on the modifications you incorporate (Mogeni, 2022).

Warm-Up Routine

Complete this entire routine before beginning the workout. It should take you no more than 10 minutes.

Pilates Imprinting

1. Lie on your back and bend your knees, keeping your feet flat on your mat.
2. Inhale and exhale deeply as you consciously relax your body from head to toe, and imprint your spine into the mat one vertebra at a time.
3. Hold for 5 breaths.

Arm Reach and Pull

1. Start out standing with your feet hip-width apart.
2. Extend your arms in front of you and reach, feeling the stretch in your shoulders.
3. Now swing your arms behind you and extend them, feeling your shoulder blades coming together.
4. Keep your breathing constant and deep as you repeat for 10 reps.

Pelvic Thrust

1. Start by lying on your mat with your palms facing the floor and your feet flat on the mat with your knees bent.
2. Engage your core and slowly lift your pelvis off the mat. Maintain a straight line from your pelvis to your shoulders as you hold for three breaths.
3. Return to the starting position and complete 10 reps.

Wall Roll-Down

1. Start with your back against a wall, with your palms on the wall and your legs extended out in front of you.
2. Nod your head downward as you roll your spine one vertebra at a time. Maintain deep breathing.
3. Slowly return to the starting position and complete five reps.

Swan Prep

1. Start out lying down on your mat.
2. Bend your elbows and raise your upper body off your mat, keeping your core engaged. Lengthen your spine and keep your neck straight.
3. Slowly lower back to the starting position.
4. Complete 10 reps.

Spine Stretch

1. Start by sitting up straight with your legs extended in front of you.
2. Raise your arms overhead and bring your body forward to form a C-shape with your spine. 3. Keep your arms extended straight in front of you.
3. Raise your torso to the starting position.
4. Complete 10 reps (Soniya, 2022).

Daily Exercise Plan

Now follow the daily exercise plan outlined below, starting with strength training and finishing with flexibility exercises.

Day	Exercises
1: Full body	**Complete the following for each exercise:** - 12–15 reps - Two to three sets - Rest for one minute between exercises **Exercises:** - High lunge pose against the wall - Wall clock - Wall burpees - Wall sphinx pose - Wall downward facing dog
2: Upper body	**Complete the following for each exercise:** - 12–15 reps per side - Two to three sets - Rest for one minute between exercises **Exercises:** - Wall bicycle crunches - Wall push-ups - Wall angels - Wall handstand - Wall dead bug
3: Lower body	**Complete the following for each exercise:** - 12–15 reps - Two to three sets - Rest for one minute between exercises

	Exercises:
	• Wall squats
	• Wall lean toe lifts
	• Wall mountain climbers
	• Wall bridge
	• Staff pose wall
4: Full body	**Complete the following for each exercise:**
	• 12–15 reps
	• Two to three sets
	• Rest for one minute between exercises
	Exercises:
	• Wall burpees
	• Wall sphinx pose
	• Wall downward facing dog
	• Wall sit with leg lifts
	• Wall plank
	• Wall shoulder stand
5: Upper body	**Complete the following for each exercise:**
	• 12–15 reps
	• Two to three sets
	• Rest for one minute between exercises
	Exercises:
	• Wall mountain climbers
	• Wall handstand
	• Wall dead bug
	Then complete the following for each exercise:
	• 20–25 reps
	• Two to three sets
	• Rest for one minute between exercises

	Exercises:
	- Wall mountain climbers
	- Wall push-ups
	- Wall slides
6: Lower body	**Complete the following for each exercise:**
	- 20–25 reps
	- Two to three sets
	- Rest for one minute between exercises
	Exercises:
	- Wall mountain climbers
	- Wall bridge
	- Staff pose wall
	- Wall sit
	- Wall squats
	- Side-lying wall leg lift
7: Rest day	
8: Full body	**Complete the following for each exercise:**
	- 20–25 reps
	- Two to three sets
	- Rest for one minute between exercises
	Exercises:
	- Wall sit with leg lifts
	- Wall plank
	- Wall shoulder stand
	- Legs-up-the-wall
	- High lunge pose against the wall
	- Wall half happy baby pose
9: Upper body	**Complete the following for each exercise:**
	- 20–25 reps
	- Two to three sets
	- Rest for one minute between exercises

	Exercises:
	- Wall push-ups
	- Wall slides
	- Wall bicycle crunches
	- Wall push-ups
	- Wall side plank
10: Lower body	**Complete the following for each exercise:**
	- 20–25 reps
	- Two to three sets
	- Rest for one minute between exercises
	Exercises:
	- Wall sit
	- Wall squats
	- Side-lying wall leg lift
	- Wall lunges
	- Wall bridge
	- Hamstring stretch in doorway
11: Full body	**Complete the following for each exercise:**
	- 20–25 reps
	- Two to three sets
	- Rest for one minute between exercises
	Exercises:
	- Legs-up-the-wall
	- High lunge pose against the wall
	- Wall half happy baby pose
	- Wall burpees
	- High lunge pose against the wall
	- Wall plank
	- Forward fold against wall

12: Upper body	**Complete the following for each exercise:** - 20–25 reps - Two to three sets - Rest for one minute between exercises **Exercises:** - Wall bicycle crunches - Wall push-ups - Wall side plank - Wall handstand - Wall pike push-ups
13: Lower body	**Complete the following for each exercise:** - 20–25 reps - Two to three sets - Rest for one minute between exercises **Exercises:** - Wall lunges - Wall bridge - Hamstring stretch in doorway - Wall scissor kicks - Wall squats - Wall garland pose (back to wall)
14: Rest day	
15: Full body	**Complete the following for each exercise:** - 25–30 reps - Two to three sets - Rest for one minute between exercises **Exercises:** - Wall burpees - High lunge pose against the wall - Wall plank - Forward fold against wall

	• Wall sit with leg lifts
	• Wall sphinx pose
	• Wall angels
	• Wall soleus stretch
16: Upper body	**Complete the following for each exercise:**
	• 25–30 reps
	• Two to three sets
	• Rest for one minute between exercises
	Exercises:
	• Wall handstand
	• Wall pike push-ups
	• Wall bicycle crunches
	• Wall push-ups
	• Wall Russian twists
17: Lower body	**Complete the following for each exercise:**
	• 25–30 reps
	• Two to three sets
	• Rest for one minute between exercises
	Exercises:
	• Wall scissor kicks
	• Wall squats
	• Wall garland pose (back to wall)
	• Wall bridge
	• Staff pose wall
	• Wall lunges
18: Full body	**Complete the following for each exercise:**
	• 25–30 reps
	• Two to three sets
	• Rest for one minute between exercises

	Exercises:
	- Wall sit with leg lifts
	- Wall sphinx pose
	- Wall angels
	- Wall soleus stretch
	- Legs-up-the-wall
	- Wall plank
	- Wall dead bug
	- Wall lean toe lifts
19: Upper body	**Complete the following for each exercise:**
	- 25–30 reps
	- Two to three sets
	- Rest for one minute between exercises
	Exercises:
	- Wall bicycle crunches
	- Wall push-ups
	- Wall Russian twists
	- Wall bicycle crunches
	- Wall handstand
	- Wall chest stretch
20: Lower body	**Complete the following for each exercise:**
	- 25–30 reps
	- Two to three sets
	- Rest for one minute between exercises
	Exercises:
	- Wall bridge
	- Staff pose wall
	- Wall lunges
	- Wall bridge
	- Wall camel pose with strap

21: Rest day	
22: Full body	**Complete the following for each exercise:** - 25–30 reps - Two to three sets - Rest for one minute between exercises **Exercises:** - Legs-up-the-wall - Wall plank - Wall dead bug - Wall lean toe lifts - High lunge pose against the wall - Wall half happy baby pose
23: Upper body	**Complete the following for each exercise:** - 25–30 reps - Three sets - Rest for one minute between exercises **Exercises:** - Wall bicycle crunches - Wall handstand - Wall chest stretch - Wall burpees - Wall sphinx pose
24: Lower body	**Complete the following for each exercise:** - 30–35 reps - Three sets - Rest for one minute between exercises **Exercises:** - Wall bridge - Wall camel pose with strap - High lunge pose against the wall

	- Wall slides - Wall garland pose (back to wall) - Wall bicycle crunches
25: Full body	**Complete the following for each exercise:** - 30–35 reps - Three sets - Rest for one minute between exercises **Exercises:** - Wall burpees - Wall sphinx pose - High lunge pose against the wall - Wall slides - Wall garland pose (back to wall)
26: Upper body	**Complete the following for each exercise:** - 30–35 reps - Three sets - Rest for one minute between exercises **Exercises:** - Wall bicycle crunches - Wall push-ups - Wall chest stretch - Wall pike push-ups - Wall slides
27: Lower body	**Complete the following for each exercise:** - 30–35 reps - Three sets - Rest for one minute between exercises **Exercises:** - Wall mountain climbers - Wall squats - Wall sits

	• Wall soleus stretch • Wall bridge
28: Rest day	
29: Full body	**Complete the following for each exercise:** • 30–35 reps • Three sets • Rest for one minute between exercises **Exercises:** • Wall bicycle crunches • Wall sphinx pose • Wall push-ups • Wall burpees • High lunge pose against the wall • Wall scissor kicks • Hamstring stretch in doorway
30: Full body	**Complete the following for each exercise:** • 30–35 reps • Three sets • Rest for one minute between exercises **Exercises:** • Wall burpees • Wall squats • Wall mountain climbers • Wall sphinx pose • Wall plank • Gastroc stretch on wall • Side-lying wall leg lift

Cool-Down Routine

Use the below workout to cool down after your vigorous exercises.

Child's Pose

Stretches the back and leg muscles.

1. Start on all fours ,then sink back to sit on your feet.
2. Extend your body forward so your body is completely folded over ,and rest your head on your arms.
3. Breathe deeply and hold for 10 breaths.

Reclining Butterfly Pose

Stretches the inner thighs and hips.

1. Start out lying on the floor on your back with your feet together and knees extended outward.
2. Raise your arms to be overhead or lying at your sides with palms facing up.
3. Hold this stretch for one minute, breathing deeply throughout.

Seated Forward Fold

Stretches the quadriceps.

1. Start by sitting with your legs extended in front of you.
2. Bend your body at your hips and stretch your arms outward in front of you, getting as close as you can reach toward your toes.
3. Keep your back straight as you lean forward, and hold the stretch for 20–30 seconds.

Knee to Chest Pose

Stretches the hamstrings and quadriceps.

1. Start by lying on the floor on your back with your body straight.
2. Bend one leg and hug your knee into your chest, interlacing your fingers around your knee or shin depending on your flexibility.
3. Hold for one minute, then switch sides.

Upper Body Stretch

Stretches the chest, shoulders, and back.

1. Start by sitting or standing in an upright position.
2. Interlace your fingers and bring your arms overhead so your palms are facing the ceiling.
3. Hold this stretch for one minute, then extend your arms behind you to a position that feels comfortable.
4. Hold the stretch for one minute.

Sew

Stretches the spinal muscles.

1. Start sitting with your legs extended outward, wider than shoulder-width apart.
2. Extend your arms outward, then twist your body, reaching one arm toward the opposite leg, getting as close as you can to your toes.
3. Alternate sides, holding each side for a few seconds.
4. Complete three to four reps on each side.

Together, these stretches target all the muscles you will have been using throughout the workout routines, so ensure you do them every day you exercise, or any other days when you feel muscle strain or tension (Cronkleton, 2019).

Track Your Progress

Use the table below to mark your progress as you complete the program. If you miss a day, don't worry! Just pick up where you left off.

Tracker						
	1	2	3	4	5	6
	7	8	9	10	11	12
	13	14	15	16	17	18
	19	20	21	22	23	24
	25	26	27	28	29	30

Use the table below to record any comments or observations from each day.

Observations
1
2
3
4
5
6

7	
8	
9	
10	
11	
12	
13	
14	
15	
16	
17	
18	
19	
20	
21	
22	
23	
24	

25	
26	
27	
28	
29	
30	

You can adjust the workouts as you see fit depending on where you are on your journey and how you feel. Always listen and respond to your body, and don't overexert yourself. As stated previously, rest days are very important and should be recorded too as progress on your path, which is why they are included in the 30-day challenge. Also, remember to stay hydrated throughout the workout routines; always have a water bottle nearby and increase your overall water intake throughout the day.

My sincere hope is that by the end of the 30-day challenge, exercising daily will have become part of your lifestyle to maintain your health and fitness; not a one-time fad, but a lifestyle change.

I Want to Hear Your Success Stories!

There's nothing more heartwarming than hearing about how other women have transformed their lives by taking their fitness into their own hands. This is your chance to share yours – and inspire others while you're at it!

Simply by sharing your honest opinion of this book and a little about your own journey with a review on Amazon, you'll inspire new readers to get started on their own routines.

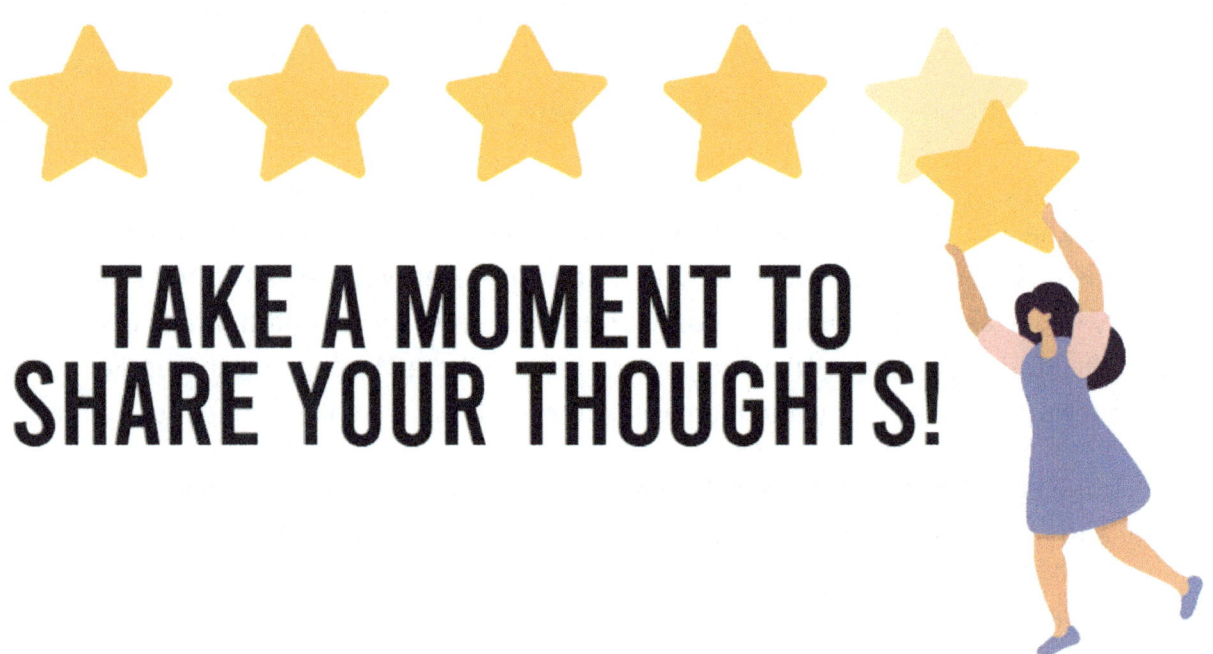

Thank you so much for your support. I can't wait to hear your story!

CONCLUSION

I hope you have found this book to be a comprehensive guide to wall Pilates through the explanations and guidance throughout. The key components to remember going forward are that your ability will improve with practice, and that your main focus should always be your form and precision throughout the exercises. Also remember the core principles of Pilates and remind yourself of them as often as you need to, making them ingrained in your mind so you can harness the full benefits of each of the workouts outlined in this book.

Hopefully, this will also encourage you to explore other forms of Pilates, as it truly is an all-encompassing form of exercise that will leave you with a stronger and more flexible body. We will finish off by considering the real-life example of a woman who used Pilates to transform her health and physical well-being and, thereby, her life.

Be Inspired: Rachel Cooke's Story

British journalist and writer Rachel Cooke accredits Pilates as one of the main things that helped her alleviate the back pain she had suffered from for years. Her pain was debilitating to the point that she could barely do any normal activities of daily life and was constantly in and out of the hospital in search of a solution. Finally, she visited a physiotherapist, who advised her to try Pilates as it had helped many others in a situation similar to hers. She reluctantly agreed to give it a shot and soon found herself attending a class run by Melanie Christou, a former dancer who herself had dealt with her back pain through Pilates.

In an article she wrote for *The Guardian*) Cooke, 2019), Rachel admits she felt embarrassed in some of the poses, and she found some exercises quite challenging. But she persisted. She attended two classes per week religiously for three years, and the changes she observed surprised her. Not only did her strength and muscle definition improve, but so did her posture and general capabilities. In addition, she felt her mental well-being improved too, and she generally had more energy and improved pelvic floor health.

She acknowledges that the changes did not come overnight, but took time and concerted effort. As previously stated, Pilates has to become part of your lifestyle, and you should also establish some longer-term goals for your health and wellness. This is not to say you will only see changes after years of practice; even after a few weeks (such as with the 30-day challenge) you will start to see changes and feel different.

Hopefully, like Rachel, you will grow to love and enjoy Pilates and harness the great things it can add to your life.

Until we meet again in the next guide, inhale, exhale, and keep on doing wall Pilates!

REFERENCES

About Pilates. (n.d.). Pilates Foundation. https://www.pilatesfoundation.com/pilates/the-history-of-pilates/

Ackler, M. (2023, July 28). *What is wall Pilates?* Pilates Anytime. https://www.pilatesanytime.com/blog/equipment/what-is-wall-pilates

Bell, J. (2022, May 13,). *Wall clocks how to: The best way to stretch your upper body.* Jen Bell Yoga. https://jenbellyoga.com/blog/wall-clocks-the-best-way-to-stretch-your-upper-body/

Bell, K. (2023, June 8). *Celebrities & athletes who swear by Pilates.* Katie Bell Physio. https://katiebellphysio.com/celebrities-athletes-who-swear-by-pilates/

Berra, Y. (n.d.). *Yogi Berra quotes.* Goodreads. https://www.goodreads.com/quotes/23616-if-you-don-t-know-where-you-are-going-you-ll-end

The best way to wall handstand for beginners. (n.d.). SummerFunFitness. https://summerfunfitness.com/the-best-way-to-wall-handstand-for-beginners/

Bona. (2023, August 27). *5 benefits of wall Pilates.* Network News. https://www.citizen.co.za/network-news/lifestyle/2023/08/27/5-benefits-of-wall-pilates/

Burritt, T. (2016, July 7). *Five basic principles of Pilates.* WellFit4EVER Pilates. https://wellfit4ever.com/five-basic-principles-pilates/

C, I. (2023, September 5). *Is it possible to get in shape at home without equipment?* Longevity. Technology. https://longevity.technology/lifestyle/is-it-possible-to-get-in-shape-at-home-without-equipment/

Camel pose with strap and wall steps. (2023). Tummee. https://www.tummee.com/yoga-poses/camel-pose-with-strap-and-wall/steps

Capritto, A. (2020, December 27). *How to do wall angels: Proper form, variations, and common mistakes.* Verywell Fit. https://www.verywellfit.com/how-to-do-wall-angels-techniques-benefits-variations-5090729

Chalicha, E. (2022, May 15). *High knees benefits, muscles worked, and how to.* BetterMe. https://betterme.world/articles/high-knees-benefits/

Chest stretch against wall: High. (n.d.). Exer-Pedia. https://exer-pedia.com/exercise/chest-stretch-against-wall-high/

Choosing the right Pilates mat. (2017, June 6). Mad-HQ. https://www.mad-hq.com/pilates-blogs/choosing-pilates-mat

Cooke, R. (2019, December 1). 'Pilates-changed-my-life' stories are annoying… but it did. *The Guardian.* https://www.theguardian.com/lifeandstyle/2019/dec/01/pilates-took-me-from-crippling-back-pain-to-amazing-health

Cronkleton, E. (2019, December 17). *16 cooldown exercises* you can do after any workout. Healthline. https://www.healthline.com/health/exercise-fitness/cooldown-exercises

Cronkleton, E. (2020, November 23). *How to do a legs-up-the-wall pose.* Healthline. https://www.healthline.com/health/exercise-fitness/legs-up-the-wall

Daisy. (2021, June 24). *Wall bridge | Illustrated exercise guide.* Spotebi. https://www.spotebi.com/exercise-guide/wall-bridge/

Davidson, K., & Davis, N. (202, May 30). *Wall pushup variations for a strong chest, shoulders, and back.* Healthline. https://www.healthline.com/health/fitness-exercise/wall-pushups

Edna, T. (2019, July 24). *Pilates: What to wear & the equipment you need.* The Sports Edit. https://thesportsedit.com/blogs/news/heres-what-to-wear-to-pilates

Evers, C. (2021, October 21). *How to do side-lying hip abductions: Proper form, variations, and common mistakes.* Verywell Fit. https://www.verywellfit.com/side-lying-hip-abductions-techniques-benefits-variations-4783963

Feiereisen, S., & Milbrand, L. (2023, October 17). *37 motivational exercise quotes to get you through (or to) your next workout.* Real Simple. https://www.realsimple.com/health/fitness-exercise/exercise-quotes

Fuhr, L. (2012, September 20). *The top 3 exercises for toned and trim thighs.* Popsugar. https://www.popsugar.com/fitness/best-exercises-thighs-25061710

Gastrocnemius stretches. (n.d.). David Redfern Surgery. https://www.davidredfernsurgery.com/gastrocstretches

Gracia, Z. (2023, October 26). *The beginner's wall plank guide for toned abs.* BetterMe. https://betterme.world/articles/wall-plank/

Guest, J. (n.d.). *Judith Guest quote. In: Guiding principles quotes.* AZ Quotes. https://www.azquotes.com/quotes/topics/guiding-principles.html

Harris-Ray, N. (n.d.). *What to know about Pilates during pregnancy.* WebMD. https://www.webmd.com/fitness-exercise/what-to-know-pilates-during-pregnancy

Healthwise Staff. (2022, November 9). *Hamstring stretch in doorway.* MyHealth.Alberta.ca. https://myhealth.alberta.ca/Health/pages/conditions.aspx?hwid=hw208009

High lunge arms extended forward with foot at wall. (n.d.). Tummee.https://www.tummee.com/yoga-poses/high-lunge-arms-extended-forward-with-foot-at-wall

High lunge pose hands wall. (n.d.). Tummee.com. https://www.tummee.com/yoga-poses/high-lunge-pose-hands-wall

Higuera, V. (2020, November 23). Health benefits of the happy baby pose (ananda balasana). Healthline. https://www.healthline.com/health/happy-baby-pose

History and origins of Pilates & the Pilates reformer. (2014, January 6). Pilates Central. https://www.pilatescentral.co.uk/history-origins-pilates/

How the Pilates mind–body connection works for you. (n.d.). Evergreen Rehab & Wellness. https://evergreenclinic.ca/how-the-pilates-mind-body-connection-works-for-you/

How the Pilates mind–body connection works for you. (2022, June 22). Frame. https://www.framefitness.com/blog/news/how-the-pilates-mind-body-connection-works-for-you

How to choose a mat for Pilates. (n.d.). Seek Solitude. https://www.seeksolitude.com.au/blogs/journal/how-to-choose-a-mat-for-pilates

How to do a wall slide: A Hinge Health guide. (n.d.). Hinge Health. https://www.hingehealth.com/resources/articles/wall-slides/

How to do sphinx pose in yoga. (2023, November 10). EverydayYoga.com. https://www.everydayyoga.com/blogs/guides/how-to-do-sphinx-pose-in-yoga

Hughes, L. (2023, September 3). *The benefits of wall Pilates for the body and mind.* Prime Women. https://primewomen.com/wellness/fitness/benefits-of-wall-pilates-for-the-body-and-mind/

Jacob, V. (2020, October 17). *Pilates expert Vesna Jacob list out precautions to take while doing Pilates.* Onlymyhealth. https://www.onlymyhealth.com/pilates-expert-listing-precautions-to-take-while-doing-pilates-1602933892

Jordan, M. (n.d.). *Michael Jordan quote. In: Fundamentals quotes.* AZ Quotes. https://www.azquotes.com/quotes/topics/fundamentals.html

Kamau, C. (2023, October 26). *Wall crunches: A simple guide to on how to do them.* BetterMe. https://betterme.world/articles/wall-crunches/

Keleher, N. (n.d.). *Shoulderstand using a wall.* Sensational Yoga Poses. https://www.sensational-yoga-poses.com/shoulderstand-using-a-wall.html

Kester, S. (2020, October 23). *Toe raises for strength and balance.* Healthline. https://www.healthline.com/health/toe-raises

Ladda, A. M., Lebon, F., & Lotze, M. (2021). Using motor imagery practice for improving motor performance – A review. *Brain and Cognition*, 150(10), 105705. https://doi.org/10.1016/j.bandc.2021.105705

MasterClass. (2021, August 11). *Wall handstand exercise guide: How to master wall handstands.* https://www.masterclass.com/articles/wall-handstand-guide

Menzies, R. (2021, August 10). *What you need to know about doing Pilates during pregnancy.* Healthline. https://www.healthline.com/health/fitness/pilates-during-pregnancy

The mind body connection: Key elements in Pilates, part 3. (n.d.). Embody Movement Pilates Studio. https://embodymovementpilates.com/the-mind-body-connection-key-elements-in-pilates-part-3/

Mogeni, R. (2022, March 212). *21 days workout schedule for total body transformation.* BetterMe. https://betterme.world/articles/21-days-workout-schedule/

Morris, M. (2023, January 31). *How to do a handstand on the wall.* WikiHow. https://www.wikihow.com/Do-a-Handstand-on-the-Wall

Mukhwana, J. (2023a, October 26). *20 wall Pilates benefits: You'll wish you knew about these sooner!* BetterMe. https://betterme.world/articles/wall-pilates-benefits/

Mukhwana, J. (2023b, October 26). *Wall Pilates FAQ: Answers from the experts.* BetterMe. https://betterme.world/articles/wall-pilates-faq/

Munuhe, N. (2023a, October 26). *Master the wall squat exercise in 6 easy steps.* BetterMe. https://betterme.world/articles/wall-squat/

Munuhe, N. (2023b, October 26). *Why is wall Pilates so effective?* BetterMe. https://betterme.world/articles/why-is-wall-pilates-so-effective/

Nguyen, J. (2014, June 4). *How to do half-dog on the wall.* DoYou. https://www.doyou.com/how-to-do-half-dog-on-the-wall/

Ogle, M. (2020, April 13). The Pilates series of five. Verywell Fit. https://www.verywellfit.com/how-to-do-pilates-scissors-exercise-2704460

phyx. (2022, November 7). *Pilates: The 6 principles of Pilates explained.* Phyx Physio + Pilates. https://www.phyxphysio.com.au/pilates-principles/

Pilates 5 basic principles. (n.d.). Sports Rehab Consulting. https://sportsrehabconsulting.com/pilates-5-basic-principles/

Pippa's Pilates & Stretch. (2016, January 24). *Wall bridges to activate & strengthen your core, glutes, and hamstrings* [Video]. YouTube. https://www.youtube.com/watch?v=_155eedZFiU

Pizer, A. (2020, September 30). *How to do garland pose (malasana) in yoga.* Verywell Fit. https://www.verywellfit.com/garland-pose-malasana-3567079

Pizer, A. (2022, April 4). *How to do staff pose (dandasana): Proper form, variations, and common mistakes.* Verywell Fit. https://www.verywellfit.com/staff-pose-dandasana-3567120

Porter, C. (2023, May 23). *What is 'wall Pilates'? Try the trend with these 5 beginner moves.* The Upside. https://www.vitacost.com/blog/what-is-wall-pilates/

Quinn, E. (2021, October 12). *How to do single leg bridges.* Verywell Fit. https://www.verywellfit.com/single-leg-bridge-exercise-3120739

Quinn, E. (2022a, June 12). *How to do a wall sit: Proper form, variations, & common mistakes.* Verywell Fit. https://www.verywellfit.com/the-wall-sit-quad-exercise-3120741

Quinn, E. (2022b, September 27). Stretching exercises for soleus and calf muscles. Verywell Fit. https://www.verywellfit.com/calf-pull-stretching-exercises-3120313

Quirt, J. (n.d.). *5 variations of uttanasana (it's more than a hamstring stretch).* Yoga International. https://yogainternational.com/article/view/variations-of-uttanasana/

Romine, S. (2020, June 23). Bored with push-ups? *Try the pike push-up.* Greatist. https://greatist.com/health/pike-pushups

Schwarzenegger, A. (n.d.). Arnold Schwarzenegger quotes. BrainyQuote. https://www.brainyquote.com/quotes/arnold_schwarzenegger_116694

Sindhu, P. V. (n.d.). *P. V. Sindhu quotes.* BrainyQuote. https://www.brainyquote.com/authors/p-v-sindhu-quotes

Soniya. (2022, May 17). *6 best warm-up exercises you must do before Pilates mat workouts.* Sportskeeda. https://www.sportskeeda.com/health-and-fitness/6-best-warm-up-exercises-to-do-before-pilates-mat-workouts

Stattman, D. (2016, October 21). *The burpee variation that's twice as hard on your abs.* Men's Health. https://www.menshealth.com/fitness/a19530343/wall-ball-burpee/

Strength training quotes. (n.d.). AZ Quotes. https://www.azquotes.com/quotes/topics/strength-training.html

The 10 principles of Pilates (2020, December 3). Nesta Certified. https://www.nestacertified.com/the-10-principles-of-pilates/

30 day challenge quotes and sayings. (n.d.). SearchQuotes. https://www.searchquotes.com/search/30_Day_Challenge/

Turnquist, C. (n.d.). *The four S's of Pilates.* Providence Pilates Center. https://www.providencepilatescenter.com/blog/the-four-ss-of-pilates

Von Oech, R. (n.d.). *Top 25 Roger Von Oech quotes.* QuoteFancy. https://quotefancy.com/roger-von-oech-quotes

Waehner, P. (2022, November 25). *How to do lunges: Proper form, variations, and common mistakes.* Verywell Fit. https://www.verywellfit.com/how-to-lunge-variations-modifications-and-mistakes-1231320

Wall bridges. (n.d.). Hybrid Calisthenics. https://www.hybridcalisthenics.com/wall-bridges

Wall lean toe raises. (n.d.). Rehab Hero. https://www.rehabhero.ca/exercise/wall-lean-toe-raises

Wall sphinx pose. (n.d.). Tummee https://www.tummee.com/yoga-poses/wall-sphinx-pose

Ward, T. (2019, January 20). Pilates dos & donts: How to have a safe & effective workout every time! Freshly Centered. https://www.freshlycentered.com/2019/01/pilates-dos-donts-how-to-have-a-safe-effective-workout-every-time/

Warwood, E. (202, May 19). *How to do a Russian twist to really fire up the core, according to trainers.* Women's Health. https://www.womenshealthmag.com/fitness/a26011033/russian-twist/

WebMD Editorial Contributor. (n.d.). *Health benefits of exercise.* WebMD. https://www.webmd.com/fitness-exercise/health-benefits-exercise

What is the mind-body connection in Pilates? (2018, November 5). JS Mind Body Pilates. https://www.jsmindbodypilates.com.au/blog/what-is-the-mind-body-connection

Williams, L. (2021, August 9). *How to do the dead bug exercise.* Verywell Fit. https://www.verywellfit.com/how-to-do-the-dead-bug-exercise-4685852

Yetman, D. (2020, November 10). The benefits of a side plank and how to do it safely. Healthline. https://www.healthline.com/health/side-plank

Shinners, Rebecca, and Elizabeth Berry. "101 Motivational Quotes About

Exercise From Famous Athletes." Woman's Day. Last modified November

19, 2022. https://www.womansday.com/health-fitness/g2318/healthy-

lifestyle-quotes/.

Made in the USA
Las Vegas, NV
04 May 2024

89532726R20070